the power of
yoga

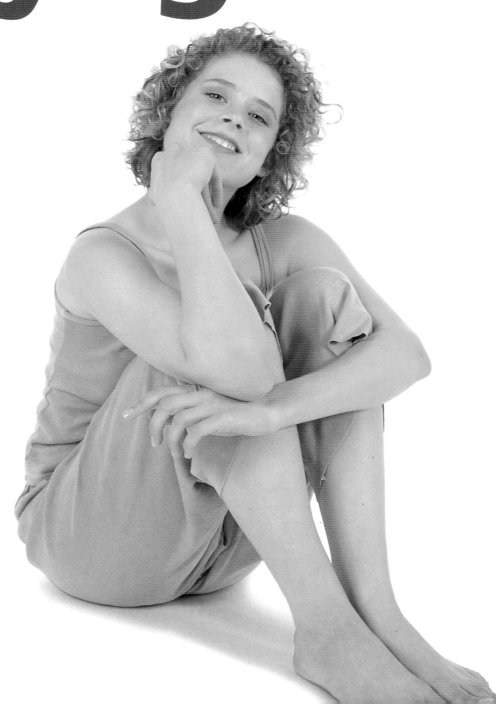

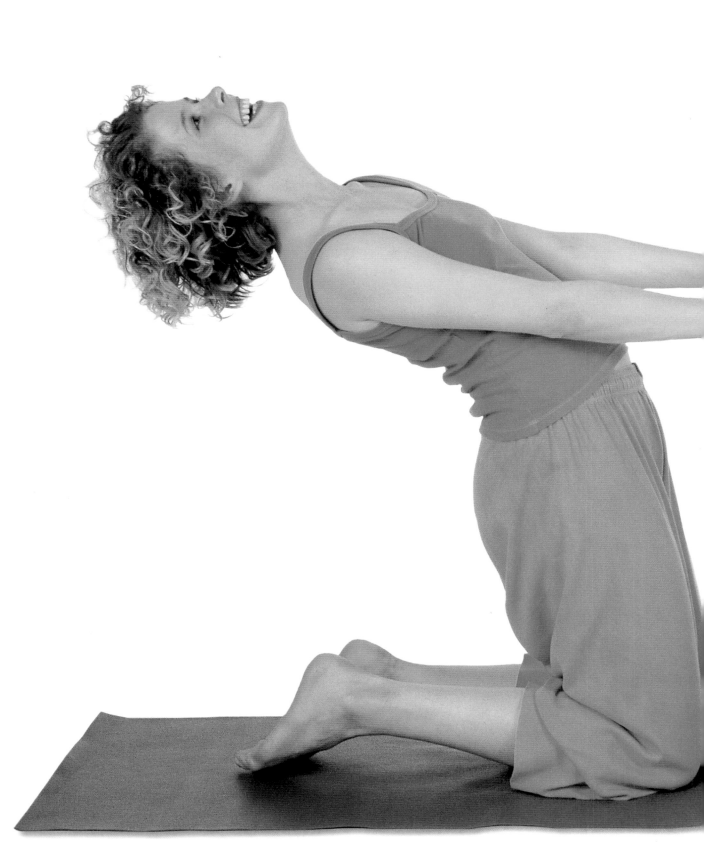

the power of
yoga

Vimla Lalvani

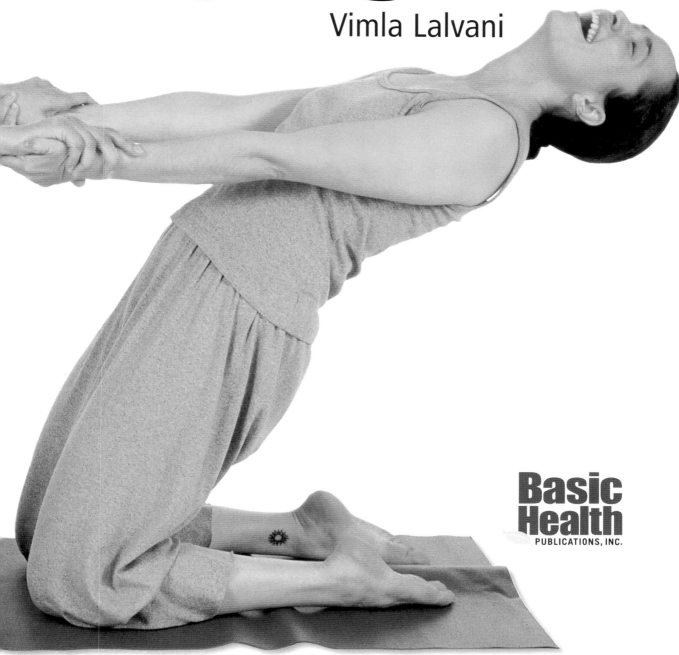

Basic Health
PUBLICATIONS, INC.

First published in North America in 2004 by Basic Health Publications, Inc.
First published 2003 in Great Britain under the title THE POWER OF YOGA by Hamlyn (an imprint, part of) Octopus Publishing Group Ltd
2-4 Heron Quays, Docklands, London E14 4JP

Text © The American Beauty Bar Ltd

Copyright © 2003 Octopus Publishing Group Limited

Basic Health Publications, Inc.
8200 Boulevard East
North Bergen, NJ 07047
1-800-575-8890

ISBN: 1-59120-117-9

Printed in China

10 9 8 7 6 5 4 3 2 1

CONTENTS

How to use this book	6
Introduction	**8**
Yoga menus	8
What is yoga?	14
Types of yoga	16
Ayurveda & yoga	18
Where & when to practice	24
Posture	26
Breathing	28
Salute to the sun	30
✔ **Yoga for exercise**	**40**
Warm-up	42
Triangle	52
Warrior 1	54
Warrior 2	56
Back bend	58
Leg lift	60
Sitting balance	64
One-arm balance	68
Letter T	72
Jet	74
Spinal twist 1	76
Breathe & relax 1	78
FACE & THROAT	
Fish	82
NECK & SHOULDERS	
Shoulder release	84
UPPER ARMS	
Push-ups	86
CHEST	
Camel	88
ABDOMEN	
Stomach stretches	90
WAIST	
Side stretch 1	92
BUTTOCKS	
Locust	94

✔ **Yoga for health** **96**
RESPIRATION
   Breathing with arms 98
   Energy booster 100
DIGESTION
   Modified bow 102
BACK PAIN
   Cat 104
   Back twist 106
NECK & SHOULDER PAIN
   Shoulder shrugs 108
   Head rolls 110
WOMEN'S PROBLEMS
   Cobra 112
   Shoulder stand 114
METABOLISM
   Plough 116
CIRCULATION & HEART
   Side stretch 2 120
   Deep lunge balance 122

✔ **Yoga for stress-relief**
  & relaxation **124**
  Balancing workout 126
  Tree 134
  Standing bow 136
  Wheel 138
  Lying flat twist 140
  Rabbit 142
  Dog 144
  Spinal twist 2 146
  Spinal twist 3 150
  Breathe & relax 2 152
  Rejuvenation 154
  Nerve soother 156
  Deep relaxation 158

✔ **Yoga for the mind & spirit 160**
  Meditation in motion 162
  Horse 172
  Elephant 174
  Lion 176
  Leg kicks 178
  Circles 180
  Pranayama 182
  Candle gazing 184
  Visualization 186

Index 188
Acknowledgments 192

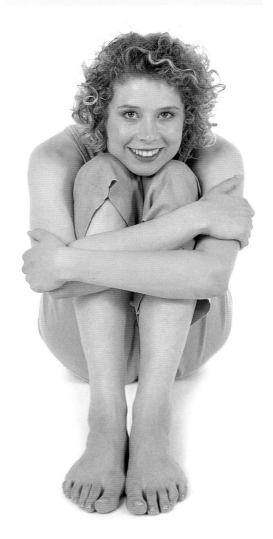

HOW TO USE THIS BOOK

The Power of Yoga is divided into 5 main sections: Introduction, Yoga for exercise, Yoga for health, Yoga for stress-relief & relaxation and Yoga for the mind & spirit.

The **Introduction** explains what yoga is and how it works, and introduces the basic techniques of posture, breathing, and the Salute to the sun. It also contains a series of yoga menus, which give suggestions for exercises to suit particular health problems or exercise needs.

Yoga for exercise contains a warm-up routine and exercises designed to improve your general fitness levels and work on particular fitness requirements, such as toning stomach muscles.

The routines in **Yoga for health** both improve your general health and well-being and work on specific health needs such as digestive ailments, back pain, and gynecological problems.

Yoga for stress-relief & relaxation contains exercises designed to help cope with the stresses of modern life and achieve natural balance and harmony.

The final chapter, **Yoga for the mind & spirit**, provides routines that help to concentrate the mind and clear it of mental clutter and introduces basic techniques for meditation.

Introductions explain how yoga exercises can help with particular health and fitness areas.

Step-by-step pictures and text are designed to lead gently through the routines.

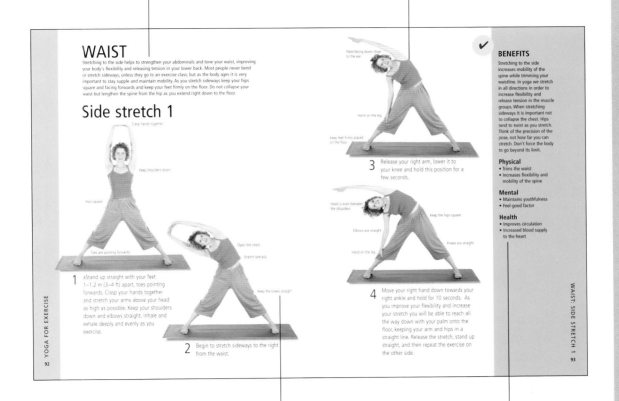

WAIST

Stretching to the side helps to strengthen your abdominals and tone your waist, improving your body's flexibility and releasing tension in your lower back. Most people never bend or stretch sideways, unless they go to an exercise class, but as the body ages it is very important to stay supple and maintain mobility. As you stretch sideways keep your hips square and facing forwards and keep your feet firmly on the floor. Do not collapse your waist but lengthen the spine from the hip as you extend right down to the floor.

Side stretch 1

Clasp hands together

Keep shoulders down

Hips square

Toes are pointing forwards

Stretch laterally

Open the chest

Keep the knees straight

1 aStand up straight with your feet 1–1.2 m (3–4 ft) apart, toes pointing forwards. Clasp your hands together and stretch your arms above your head as high as possible. Keep your shoulders down and elbows straight. Inhale and exhale deeply and evenly as you exercise.

2 Begin to stretch sideways to the right from the waist.

Palm facing down close to the ear

Hand on the leg

Keep feet firmly placed on the floor

3 Release your right arm, lower it to your knee and hold this position for a few seconds.

Head is even between the shoulders

Elbows are straight

Hand on the leg

Keep the hips square

Knees are straight

4 Move your right hand down towards your right ankle and hold for 10 seconds. As you improve your flexibility and increase your stretch you will be able to reach all the way down with your palm onto the floor, keeping your arm and hips in a straight line. Release the stretch, stand up straight, and then repeat the exercise on the other side.

BENEFITS

Stretching to the side increases mobility of the spine while trimming your waistline. In yoga we stretch in all directions in order to increase flexibility and release tension in the muscle groups. When stretching sideways it is important not to collapse the chest. Hips tend to twist as you stretch. Think of the precision of the pose, not how far you can stretch. Don't force the body to go beyond its limit.

Physical
• Trims the waist
• Increases flexibility and mobility of the spine

Mental
• Maintains youthfulness
• Feel-good factor

Health
• Improves circulation
• Increased blood supply to the heart

Pointers indicate particular things to watch out for that will help you get the most out of the routines.

The Benefits panel explains the routine's effectiveness in all areas of fitness and health, both physical and mental.

INTRODUCTION
Yoga menus

As well as increasing overall fitness and well-being, yoga exercises can be used for specific purposes, for example, toning muscles, relieving localized aches and pains, or alleviating stress-related disorders. The menus over the next few pages offer suggestions for combinations of beneficial yoga exercises. They are arranged by body part, starting with the head and finishing with the feet. So, for instance, exercises that will help migraine sufferers will be found under "head & face" and those that are good for gynecological problems are found under "pelvic region."

Body part	Posture	Pages
HEAD & FACE		
Facial muscles	Fish	82–83
Stress-relief	Breathing with arms	98–99
Concentration	*Pranayama*	182–183
	Candle gazing	184–185
	Visualization	186–187
	Tree	134–135
	Standing bow	136–137
	Horse	172–173
	Lion	176–177
Headaches	Dog	144–145
Migraine	Rabbit	142–143
	Nerve soother	156–157
	Deep relaxation	158–159
Insomnia	Rabbit	142–143
Master hormone	Dog	144–145

NECK & SHOULDERS

Stiff neck	Shoulder release	84–85
	Head rolls	110–111
Shoulder tension	Shoulder release	84–85
	Breathing with arms	98–99
	Shoulder shrugs	108–109
	Shoulder stand	114–115
Whiplash	Shoulder shrugs	108–109
	Head rolls	110–111

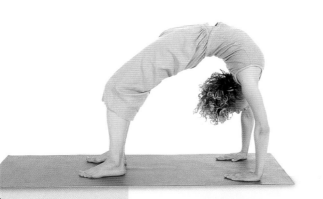

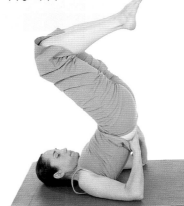

ARMS

Muscle definition	One-arm balance	68–71
	Push-ups	86–87
	Dog	144–145
Upper & lower arms	Triangle	52–53
	One-arm balance	68–71
	Push-ups	86–87
	Cobra	112–113
	Dog	144–145
	Wheel	138–139
	Rejuvenation	154–155
Elbow joint problems	One-arm balance	68–71
	Letter T	72–73
	Spinal twist 1	76–77
Wrist problems	Meditation in motion	162–171
	Cobra	112–113

CHEST

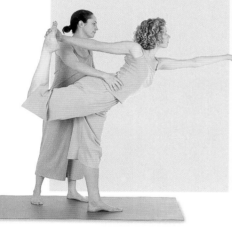

Pectoral muscles

Salute to the sun	30–39
Back bend	58–59
Jet	74–75
Camel	88–89
Energy booster	100–101
Cobra	112–113
Standing bow	136–137
Wheel	138–139

Heart & circulation

Salute to the sun	30–39
Warm-up	42–51
Warrior 2	56–57
Letter T	72–73
Side stretch 1	92–93
Side stretch 2	120–121
Balancing workout	126–133
Deep lunge balance	122–123
Elephant	174–175

BACK

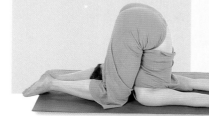

Lower back pain

Locust	94–95
Back twist	106–107
Cobra	112–113

Upper back pain

Plough	116–119
Lying flat twist	140–141
Rabbit	142–143
Dog	144–145
Spinal twist 2	146–149

Waist

Triangle	52–53
Warrior 2	56–57
Spinal twist 1	76–77
Side stretch 1	92–93
Balancing workout	126–133

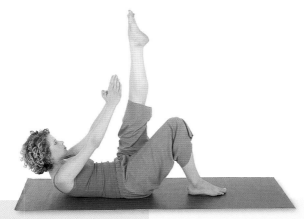

ABDOMEN

Stomach muscles	Leg lift	60–63
	Sitting balance	64–67
	Stomach stretches	90–91
	Shoulder stand	114–115
	Plough	116–119
	Lying flat twist	140–41
	Spinal twist 3	150–51
	Leg kicks	178–179
Digestive disorders	Locust	94–95
	Modified bow	102–103
	Cat	104–105
	Cobra	112–113
Digestive hormones	Warrior 1	54–55
	Jet	74–75
	Spinal twist 1	76–77
	Rabbit	142–143
	Spinal twist 2	146–149

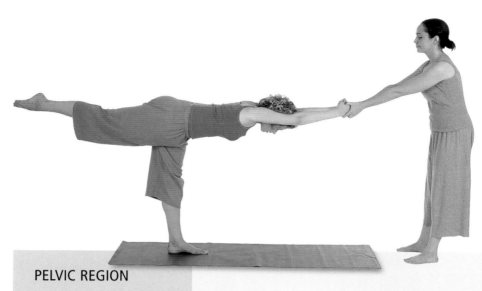

PELVIC REGION

Gynecological problems	Cobra	112–113
	Shoulder stand	114–115
Cramps	Plough	116–119
	Dog	144–145
Pregnancy	Breathe & relax 1	78–81
	Breathe & relax 2	152–153
	Nerve soother	156–157
Buttocks	Back bend	58–59
	One-arm balance	68–71
	Letter T	72–73
	Jet	74–75
	Locust	94–95
	Modified bow	102–103
	Cat	104–105
	Balancing workout	126–133
	Standing bow	136–137
	Wheel	138–139
	Rejuvenation	154–155

LEGS

Thighs	Warrior 1	54–55
	Warrior 2	56–57
	Camel	88–89
	Deep lunge balance	122–123
	Horse	172–173
	Elephant	174–175
	Leg kicks	178–179
	Circles	180–181
Knees	Triangle	52–53
	Back bend	58–59
	Leg lift	60–63
	Camel	88–89
	Tree	134–135
Feet & ankles	Triangle	52–53
	Warrior 1	54–55
	Warrior 2	56–57
	Back bend	58–59
	One-arm balance	68–71
	Letter T	72–73
	Push-ups	86–87
	Tree	134–135
	Standing bow	136–137

What is yoga?

Yoga is an ancient science, developed thousands of years ago, that teaches us how to live life successfully. It is not a religion but a living philosophy of life that gives us the power to change our lives and teaches us how to find a new vision, a new way of looking at the universe and ourselves—to find inner peace in a chaotic world and compassion that will radiate and permeate in every aspect of the Self.

What does the word yoga mean?

The word "yoga" derives from Sanskrit and means the union of mind, body, and spiritual self. It comes from the ancient texts of the *Vedas*, which were written at least 5,000 years ago. It is a discipline that unifies all aspects of the whole person, and integrates the mental, physical, emotional, and spiritual nature of every human being. The natural state of man is to be balanced and be in harmony with nature, but the trials and tribulations of modern living constantly throw us off balance.

Yoga and inner balance

Yoga restores balance and harmony to the system and the results can be seen on both the internal and external body. Yoga is as relevant today as it was thousands of years ago. It deals with universal truths and is a practical tool for all people. With the advancement of science and its ability to test which areas of the mind and body are stimulated during yoga practice, we can now understand the ancient wisdom of the sages who developed this science all those centuries ago.

How can yoga help us?

The popularity of yoga has soared in recent years through increased interest from the media, as well as role models who testify to the benefits of yoga. Modern life is stressful, and many people are looking for alternative methods to achieve health and happiness. Most have tried many different types of fitness regimes only to find that they are easily bored and achieve no lasting results.

Yoga and fitness

With yoga, however, there are many benefits, and the results can be seen on all aspects of the mind and body. The deep stretching exercises elongate or lengthen each muscle so the physical body is toned and supple. They also improve the flexibility of the spine, and this keeps us youthful. Holding the poses for a length of time increases strength and stamina. Energy levels are increased, and this boosts morale and confidence. The specific deep-breathing exercises increase levels of oxygen in the bloodstream, which replenishes each cell and nerve in the body, thus rejuvenating all the internal organs so the system is working perfectly like a well-tuned car. Yoga works on the central nervous system so we become calm and tranquil with a positive attitude toward life. Yoga is a discipline, and when you practice yoga on a regular basis, you will see the results—an invigorated body, glowing complexion, sparkling eyes, a positive mind, and a sense of inner calm.

How does yoga work?

All yogic exercises are based on a formula of stretching, relaxation, and deep breathing. Graceful, fluid movements create strength and balance of mind, body, and spirit. The purpose of yoga is not to build muscle but to build muscle tone. The deep stretching helps to eliminate fat within the cells, reducing the appearance of cellulite. Yoga exercises build the immune system so you rarely experience such problems as the common cold. The stresses and strains of modern living take a toll on us physically and mentally, making us more vulnerable to more serious diseases, and yoga also helps to strengthen and boost the immune system so it can fight against such problems as cancer, AIDS, and heart attacks. Yoga exercises also regulate our metabolism and hormone levels.

Yoga and aging

As we age, our metabolisms slow down and many people complain about a gradual gain in weight—commonly known as middle-age spread. Yoga *asanas* keep the metabolism stable so your weight will not fluctuate, and you will be able to maintain your ideal weight. One of the main benefits of yoga is its ability to help us deal with stress. Even though we cannot switch off from the world completely, we can certainly help ourselves cope. The deep stretching exercises combined with *Pranayama* breathing reduces stress in the muscle groups. The art of relaxation reduces mental stress, relaxes the brain, and soothes the nerves.

Mind techniques

The mind techniques of visualization and meditation teach us how to empty the mind of confusing thoughts, giving clarity and stillness. When the mind is still, one can focus clearly on disturbing problems and calmly resolve the issues rationally. This applies to mundane problems or the plight of the human condition. Learning the technique of mastery over the mind brings empowerment to the human Soul.

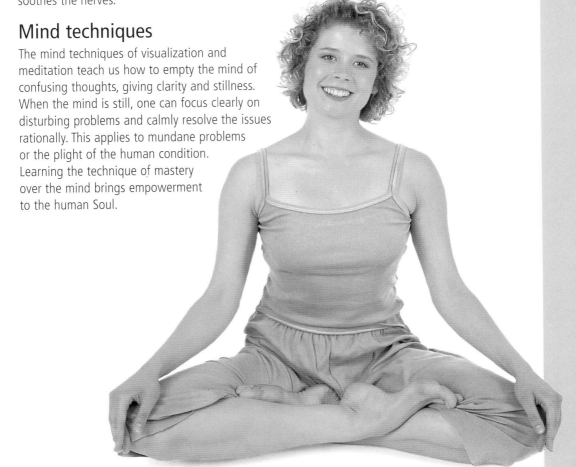

Types of yoga

All types of yoga have the same goal. The main purpose is to unite the Self with the Cosmic Universe. Different paths were documented in the *Vedas,* and they reasoned that because we are unique and different, our personalities would determine which path to follow. For best results, all paths should be considered and practiced. The 4 mental paths are *Bhakti* Yoga, *Gyana* Yoga, *Raj* Yoga, and *Karma* Yoga.

The 4 paths

When people first begin practicing yoga, they can sense that it is much more than mere exercise. The mind is learning to focus and concentrate, and the four paths achieve this in different ways. *Raj* Yoga is the study of the discipline of the mind and teaches meditation. The path of yoga is spiritual, and people who practice *Raj* Yoga usually develop a spiritual calling and use this practice to reach Nirvana—celestial bliss. To unite with the Universal Cosmos, as taught in the Hindu and Buddhist religions, is the goal of the aspirant of *Raj* Yoga. *Bhakti* Yoga is devotional in nature and deals with emotions. Chanting, prayer, and repetition of mantras transform emotional love to Divine Love. *Karma* Yoga is living life with compassion for all beings and performing good deeds for humankind. It is selfless service to benefit the world while working on a spiritual level. *Gyana* Yoga is for intellectual philosophers who study the ancient scriptures of the *Vedanta*.

Physical yoga

The one physical form of yoga is called *Hatha* Yoga, which comes under *Raj* Yoga, and is the type covered in this book. *Hatha* means the union of the sun and moon or, in modern terms, the unification of masculine and feminine energies. Every person, whether male or female, has both energies within, and the purpose of yoga is to balance these two energies so each person is in harmony with life.

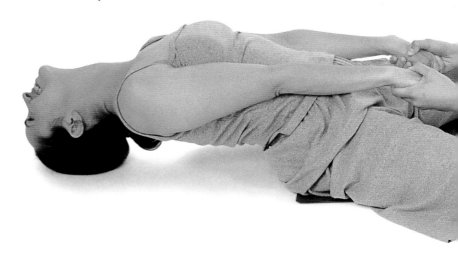

Kundalini Yoga is also a form of *Raj* Yoga. *Kundalini* Yoga has been the best-kept secret of yoga for thousands of years, known only to Hindu sages and mystics. *Kundalini* is the vital cosmic energy that lies curled like a dormant snake or serpent at the base of the spine, unless you reawaken and activate the spirit. This is done with specific yogic practices that stir the sleeping serpent, which when aroused leads to heightened consciousness that unifies one with God or universal energy. Even though there are different types of yoga, *Hatha* Yoga is the most popular. It is also called the first stage of yoga. The philosophy states that to be able to discipline your mind, you must first discipline the body.

Training the physical body to be strong, toned, and dynamic is the prime target for people who practice yoga *asanas*, or postures. Learning to calm the nervous system through the art of relaxation and visualization is the goal of many students who are learning to deal with the stresses of life. Yoga serves as a preventive measure to serious illness, but therapeutic yoga helps relieve symptoms of many common ailments that people often experience. Specific exercises for migraine, backache, arthritis, asthma, and panic attacks, to name a few, help to relieve pain and prevent the complaint recurring.

The relevance of yoga today

Many doctors today see the relevance of yoga and prescribe it for their patients in an effort to cure more serious diseases. Many new studies in leading universities and hospitals show clinical evidence of the neurological benefits of yoga to the body as a whole. Passive yoga is when the physician administers yoga postures to a person who is disabled or elderly, and doctors have found great success in reconnecting the mind and body. This technique is particularly useful for people who have been injured in accidents when their nerves have been damaged. Yoga works on the central nervous system so the mind is reactivated and sends messages to the brain that begin the rehabilitation process.

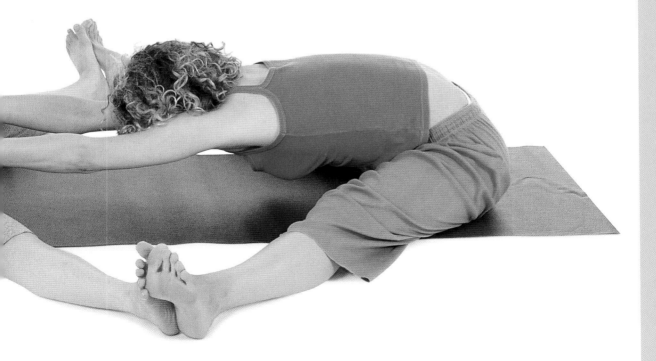

Ayurveda & yoga

There is a direct link between yoga and *Ayurveda*. They are both born from the same school of ancient literature called the *Vedas*. It says that the mental, physical, emotional, and spiritual energies of a person must be balanced and in total harmony to be in perfect health. *Ayurveda* is the medical science that treats the whole person, and yoga is the discipline that unites these energies. They work hand in hand and complement one another. Yoga is the ultimate goal to self-realization (although most of us accept that we will never reach it), and *Ayurveda* leads the path to perfect health. This medical science states that every individual is unique and each of us must therefore be viewed differently.

The three doshas

Ayurveda teaches that people are divided into three primary types according to their mental constitution, emotional responses, physical traits, and spiritual awareness, and these three will react differently to different situations. These mind-body types are called *doshas,* and it is vital to discover which you are to understand yourself better and create a life management program as specific and unique as you are. The *asanas* and *Pranayama* breathing and meditation practices appropriate for one *dosha* may not be as useful to another. No type is better than another. Each has its own strengths and weaknesses.

No one person is one type only but a combination. The predominant trait determines the *dosha*. The three *doshas* are *Vata*, *Pitta,* and *Kapha*. *Vata* controls movement or catabolism, *Pitta* controls metabolism, and *Kapha* controls structure or anabolism. To stay alive, every cell in our body has to contain all three principles. *Vata* in the body allows it to breathe, send nerve impulses to and from the brain, circulate blood, pass food through the digestive tract, and grasp ideas. *Pitta* allows it to process food, water, air, and thoughts. *Kapha* holds the cells together, forms tissues, and stimulates mental remembrance.

Prakruti

The basic constitution, the *Prakruti*, of the individual is fixed at the moment of conception. It is based on the condition in their parents' bodies and minds. The pattern is etched permanently into the genetic material and remains unchanged or unaltered during a person's lifetime. When the three *doshas* are equal in quantity, they balance each other. When they are structurally and functionally in a normal state, they maintain good health.

Even though *Prakruti* does not change, *Vikrruti*—the current state of one's health—is subject to change. When imbalances occur in the *doshas*, changes within the constitution arise, which manifest themselves as symptoms of disease.

What is your dosha?

Vata symbolizes the elements of ether + air: it literally means "wind." When balanced, it motivates creativity, speed, agility, and enthusiasm. Negative or disturbed *Vata* causes mental, nervous, and digestive disorders, including low energy and weakening of all bodily tissues. *Vata* types have the weakest build but the greatest capacity for change and adaptation in order to protect it.

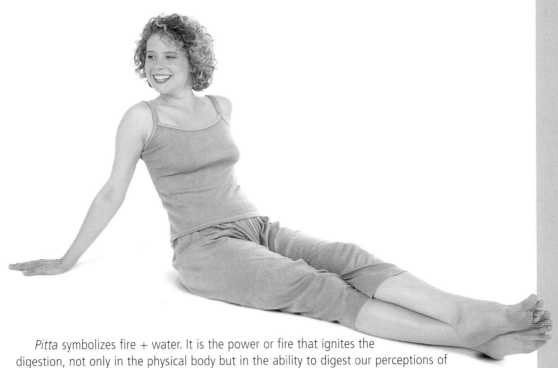

Pitta symbolizes fire + water. It is the power or fire that ignites the digestion, not only in the physical body but in the ability to digest our perceptions of the world. *Pitta* endows us with the positive traits of intelligence, courage, and vitality. Without it, we become fearful and lack motivation and decisiveness to accomplish goals. A negative *Pitta* type will build toxins that can give rise to infection and inflammation. *Pitta* types have moderate physical strength but greater mental and emotional force.

Kapha is water + earth. Simply, it means the matter or substance that sticks things together or the power of cohesion. A balanced *Kapha* endows us with emotion and feeling. This gives love, caring, devotion, loyalty, and faith, which create harmony within us as well as with others. *Kapha*'s water replenishes the tissues with nourishment. When afflicted, *Kapha* creates an abundance of excess mucus, which can lead to overweight or obesity, lung disorders, swollen glands, and an impaired immune system.

The benefits of Ayurvedic medicine

Ayurveda physicians are able to cure and prevent many different diseases using herbs, barks of trees, spices, minerals, and plant extracts. Many cures have been documented for cancer, AIDSs, heart disease, skin disorders, and mental depression. The medicine is highly effective and powerful without the side effects usually related to chemical drugs, and so the popularity of *Ayurveda* medicine is on the increase. *Ayurveda* doctors always prescribe yoga exercise as a way to balance and harmonize the *doshas*. There are specific yoga *asanas* that help to balance each *dosha*. For *Vata* types, the emphasis would be to build stamina, boost energy levels, and calm and soothe the nervous system. For *Pitta* types, the emphasis is on creating positive thinking, boosting the immune system, and detoxifying the body from harmful poisons. For *Kapha* types, the emphasis would be to rebalance hormonal levels and thyroid imbalances as well as dynamic exercises to shape and tone the body while burning calories to maintain weight.

It is important to know your particular type because it allows you to select appropriate habits and lifestyles to prevent disease. It focuses on diet, behavior, daily routine, and exercise to evolve to a more ideal state of health and personal happiness. It helps you understand yourself and others and to change your personality.

The dosha questionnaire

An individual constitution can be assessed by reading the following questionnaire. Check the characteristics listed that most accurately describe you the majority of the time. Add up the total number from the bottom of each of the columns. The *dosha* with which you share the most characteristics is your predominant constitution.

For example, if your score is V: 10, P: 6, K: 1 your predominant dosha is *Vata-Pitta*. This represents the primary *doshas* that govern your emotions, body, mind, and spirit.

VATA
Physical

Frame	thin, slender or light with prominent joints and bony contours
Height	either tall or short
Weight	light or underweight
Skin	dry, rough, brittle, creaked, dark, or brownish
Hair	rough, dry, thin, scanty, and lacks luster
Eyes	smoky sclera
Teeth	crooked
Nails	rough and brittle
Nose	bent or turned up

Functional

Appetite	variable, comes in bursts
Thirst	variable
Digestion	tendency to get constipation
Tastes/cravings	sweet, sour, salty, hot drinks, pastry, crunchy or easy-to-grab food, such as potato chips
Sleeping habits	light or interrupted with a tendency to insomnia
Body temperature	cold feet and hands, dislikes cold
Walk	walks quickly
Energy/stamina	energetic in bursts but gets exhausted quickly and has low stamina
Activity	very active and is often restless, does everything fast
Speech	talkative and speaks quickly
Financial status	poor, spends readily on trifles

Emotional

Basic traits	sensitive, highly strung, changeable, and quick to react
Positive tendencies	flexible, detached, and open
Negative tendencies	impatient, easily upset, fearful, anxious, suspicious, lacks confidence, and is nervous, but can also appear bold

Mental

Thinking	alert, restless mind, likes to communicate, scattered thinking
Learning ability	learns quickly
Memory	poor, forgets easily
Likes— colors	gray, brown, darkish, and sad
music	loud, avant-garde, and non-harmonious
cars	practical and inexpensive
furniture	unfussy and and functional, second-hand or antiques
natural world	mountains, extreme conditions

PITTA
Physical

Frame	medium, delicate; slender or roundish shape with prominent veins and tendons
Height	medium
Weight	medium
Skin	thin, smooth, warm, yellowish or in reddish color, with moles
Hair	thin, silky, straight, reddish or brownish, which tends to go gray early
Eyes	small, sharp and penetrating, gray, green, or copper-brown
Teeth	yellowish
Nails	soft, thin, and delicate
Nose	sharp

Functional

Appetite	good–excessive, becomes unbearable if not fed regularly
Thirst	excessive
Digestion	strong, quick with a tendency toward diarrhea, prone to ulcers
Tastes/cravings	sweet, bitter, astringent, cool drinks
Sleeping habits	moderate and sound, but may not go back to sleep if awakened
Body temperature	raised and always feels warm
Walk	dignified
Energy/stamina	moderate and stable
Financial status	moderately well off, likes luxury and to show off wealth

Emotional

Basic traits	strong, forceful, exuberant, feisty, or even domineering
Positive tendencies	ambitious, responsible and punctual, has good leadership and decision-making skills
Negative tendencies	prone to feelings of hatred, anger, jealousy; can be judgemental, critical, impatient, and irritable

Mental

Thinking	quick, intelligent and penetrating, with good organizational and analytical skills and powers of comprehension, likes good arguments
Learning ability	fast and precise
Memory	sharp or moderate
Speech	moderate use of words but still good, persuasive orator
Likes— colors	red, orange, yellow, and gold
music	light-baroque, such as Mozart
cars	fast, red sports models
furniture	functional yet elegant

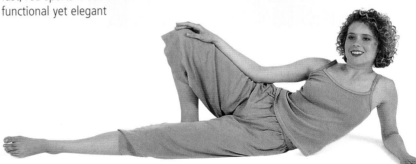

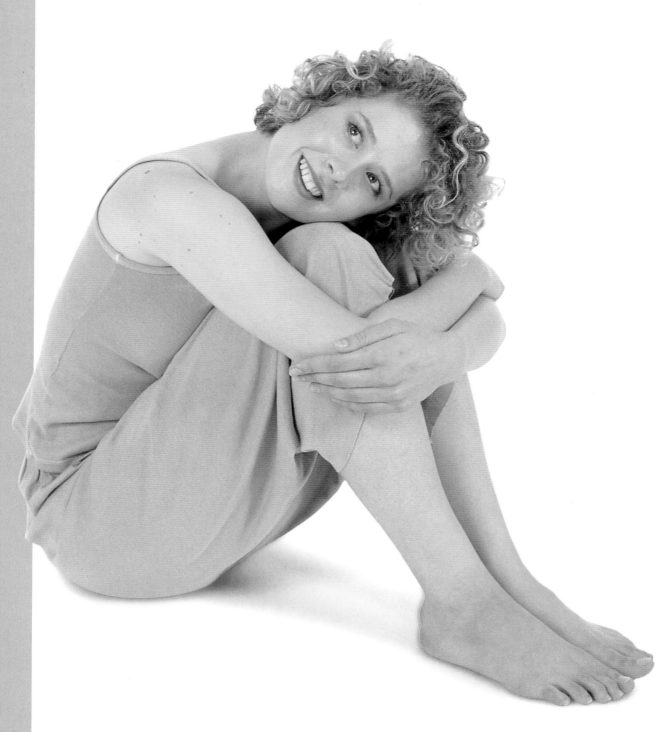

KAPHA
Physical

Frame	well-developed, stout, with a broad chest
Height	medium
Weight	heavy with a tendency toward overweight
Skin	soft, silky, oily, cold, and pale
Hair	thick, soft, abundant, dark, and wavy
Eyes	dense, black or blue, large and moist; uses them effectively
Teeth	white, regular, and attractive
Nails	soft, thick, and lustrous
Nose	well-formed

Functional

Appetite	moderate to low
Thirst	low
Digestion	slow
Tastes/cravings	pungent, bitter, and astringent foods
Sleeping habits	heavy, prolonged; has difficulties waking up
Body temperature	medium
Walk	slow, dignified, elegant
Energy/stamina	steady, high
Financial status	tends to be wealthy, good at holding on to money

Emotional

Basic traits	calm, quiet, steady, and serious
Positive tendencies	patient, kind, strong, humble, tolerant, accepting, and loyal
Negative tendencies	greedy, possessive, gets over-attached

Mental

Thinking		slow, steady, reaches well-considered conclusions
Learning		comprehension is slow but definite
Memory		good long-term memory
Activity		slow-moving, inactive, or passive
Speech		slow, with a sweet voice
Likes—	colors	light blue, light green
	furniture	heavy, elegant, expensive, stylish

Where & when to practice

In order to see the results and feel the benefits of yoga exercise, you need to practice at least three times a week. Yoga is a discipline, and as you continue to practice on a regular basis, it will become something you look forward to. As a beginner, it is easier if you choose the same time every day. It does not matter what time of the day it is, as long as there are no likely disturbances. Choose a time when you can switch yourself off from the rest of the world, away from children, telephones, and everyday noise.

Create the best environment

Find a quiet, cozy corner. Wear comfortable clothing and always try to have bare feet. In the winter months, socks are acceptable, but you will need to be careful not to slip— a non-slip yoga mat will help with this. Feet play an extremely important role in yoga exercise because the nerve endings of every organ in the body are in the feet and being barefoot allows you to connect with the earth's energy. In addition, having bare feet helps with maintaining your balance, and the toes need to grip the floor in order to maintain the challenging standing poses. It is always nice to set the mood. Turn on music that you like and switch off the telephone. It is better to practice the whole program rather than to start and stop.

Take it at your own speed

Many people feel frustrated when they first start to practice yoga. Yoga is a challenge— it is meant to be so. Take it slowly and follow at your own pace. Remember that yoga is non-competitive: It is about you and you alone and teaches you a lot about your own responses and reactions. Because of where you are mentally, physically, emotionally, and spiritually, your yoga will reflect the present state you are in. There will be some *asanas* that you will love to do and others that you will simply hate. This is quite normal. The *asanas* you hate are the ones you need to do in order to balance yourself properly. You will also find that you can do some *asanas* better on the right side and others better on the left side. This is all part of the process of balancing masculine and feminine energies within yourself. Keep an open mind.

An *asana* that you might find difficult might be very simple for the next person. Never feel discouraged. With continued practice you will surprise yourself. During my 30 years of teaching I have seen the joy and surprise of many students who achieve poses they never dreamed they could accomplish.

Every thought starts in the mind, so if you set your mind to it and challenge yourself, you will see the results for yourself. Be patient and set a series of goals for yourself. Progress is seen in various stages. Increased flexibility, strength, and stamina are the first physical attributes to change, and will be accompanied by a developing sense of inner calm. Your energy levels will increase, and you will feel invigorated. The second stage is that your concentration and focus will improve during your yoga practice, and you will feel more in control of your life. The third stage is that you will feel like a different person

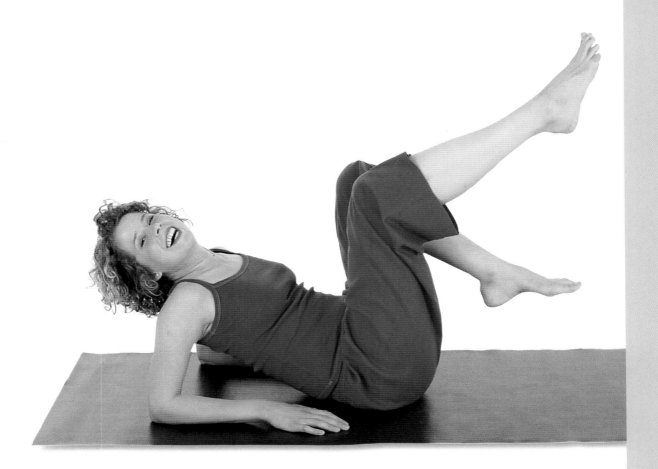

from before. You are totally integrated; all aspects of mind, body, and spiritual Self are unified. You will sense the difference immediately; you are filled with inner joy.

Yoga and lifestyle changes

Many students ask whether they need to change their diet and lifestyle. Yoga is about moderation, not about saying no. When you begin your yoga practice, you will find your equilibrium. When you are in touch with yourself, you will know what you can or cannot eat, which social habits you can continue with, and where to find moderation in all aspects of your life.

Contraindications

This book is designed for people who are in good general health; if you have any medical problems, please consult your doctor before you begin. If you are pregnant, do not attempt any inverted posture that takes your legs over your head. This can tilt the uterus and is obviously unadvisable. Do not practice yoga on a full stomach. Wait two hours after a small meal or four hours after a main meal. Many people feel nausea or dizziness when they first begin practicing yoga. This is very normal. The nausea is due to the build-up of toxins in the body. Yoga exercise releases the harmful poisons that are trapped in the system. Alcohol, smoking, prescription drugs, and pollution all contribute to a build-up of toxins. The increased intake of oxygen to the system gained through yoga can make one feel lightheaded. These two reactions pass fairly swiftly and should not put you off your exercises.

Posture

Correct posture forms the basis of all yoga exercise. Think of a string at the top of your head pulling you upward. If you are standing, make sure that the weight is evenly distributed between your toes and heels. Lift your heels and balance on your toes. If you fall forward or backward you are not in perfect posture.

This standing pose is called *Tadasana,* or Mountain Pose. You should feel strong and immovable, as a mountain would. Keep your gaze straight ahead. Lift your head up with shoulders back and chest open, and make sure that your knees are straight. In the beginning you can stand against a wall to test your alignment.

In time, you will actually feel and know that you are in perfect posture. This pose teaches balance, centering the body, and attentiveness. It looks very simple, but concentrating on every muscle focuses the mind and creates a positive attitude to life. When you stand, kneel, or sit in perfect posture, you will know and feel the difference.

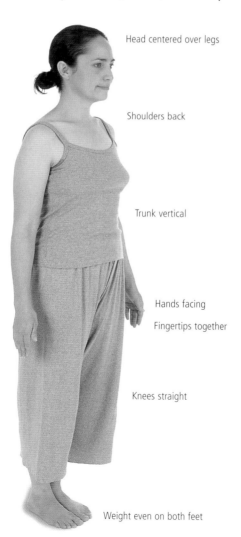

Head centered over legs

Shoulders back

Trunk vertical

Hands facing

Fingertips together

Knees straight

Weight even on both feet

1 Stand tall with your feet together and arms at your sides. Keep your eyes focused ahead and your chin level. Feel as if there is a string pulling you upward. Open your chest, and keep the shoulders down. Breathe deeply and evenly and hold for 5–7 counts. Try to turn your attention into yourself and stand as still as possible to steady the mind.

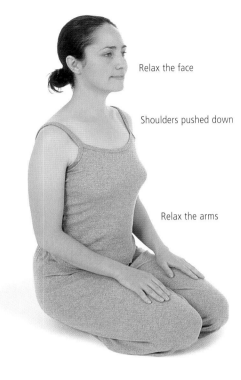

Relax the face

Shoulders pushed down

Relax the arms

2 Kneel on the floor. Place the palms facing down on to the top of the thighs. Keep the gaze ahead.

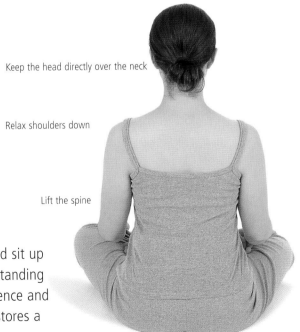

Keep the head directly over the neck

Relax shoulders down

Lift the spine

3 Cross the legs at the ankles, and sit up as tall as possible. Sitting and standing in perfect posture boost confidence and improve your appearance. It restores a positive mental attitude.

Breathing

Breath is the source of life, and yoga breathing techniques, or *Pranayama,* teach you how to tap into your energy potential. In yoga, we breathe through the nose from the diaphragm. As you inhale, the stomach extends outward, and as you exhale, the stomach contracts inward. With the increase in oxygen, each cell in the body is nourished. The increased oxygen in the blood supply replenishes and rejuvenates all the internal organs. The inhalation brings vital energy, or *prana,* to the body, and the exhalation releases toxins. Correct breathing acts as a natural tranquilizer to the system. The deeper you breathe, the calmer the mind becomes. You don't even need to think about it. It just happens automatically. Deep breathing also steadies the mind and turns your attention inward.

Most people do not know how to breathe correctly and are virtually starving the body of essential oxygen. Yoga breathing teaches you how to increase your lung capacity. Try to feel the difference between the quality of the breath between the right and left nostrils. The right is masculine energy, so it should feel warmer and louder, while the left is cooler and softer.

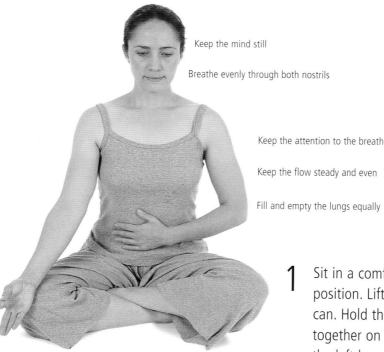

Keep the mind still

Breathe evenly through both nostrils

Keep the attention to the breath

Keep the flow steady and even

Fill and empty the lungs equally

1 Sit in a comfortable cross-legged position. Lift the spine as tall as you can. Hold the thumb and first finger together on the right hand. Place the left hand to the diaphragm or lower abdomen. Concentrate on the breath only.

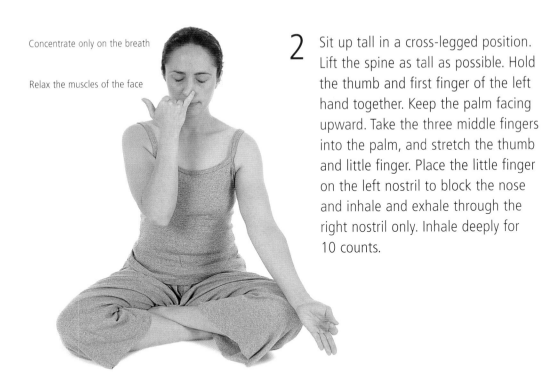

Concentrate only on the breath

Relax the muscles of the face

2 Sit up tall in a cross-legged position. Lift the spine as tall as possible. Hold the thumb and first finger of the left hand together. Keep the palm facing upward. Take the three middle fingers into the palm, and stretch the thumb and little finger. Place the little finger on the left nostril to block the nose and inhale and exhale through the right nostril only. Inhale deeply for 10 counts.

3 Change the hands so that the thumb is blocking the right nostril. Inhale and exhale for 10 counts.

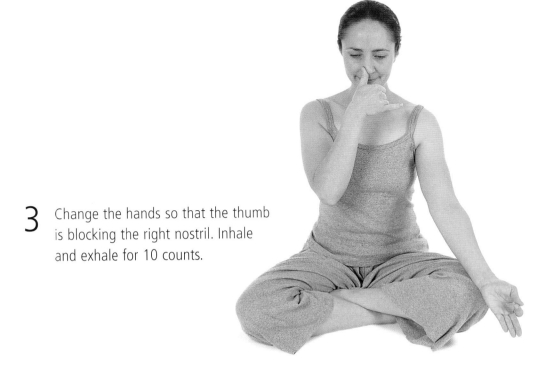

Salute to the sun

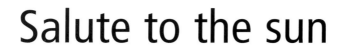

This top to toe exercise is called the yoga warm-up because it stretches and tones every muscle in the body. Combined with correct breathing, it wakes up the body and is an ideal exercise to start the day. This is a series of 19 steps and is called a *vinyasa*, with one movement flowing into another. Think of yourself as a dancer as you move from one position to the next. Try not to jerk, and keep your breath steady and flowing smoothly with the movement.

Keep elbows in line

Knees are straight

1 Stand up tall. Place your palms together in prayer position, keeping your shoulders down. Breathe normally.

Elbows straight

Arms close to ears

Head back slightly

Push hips forward and arch the back

2 Inhale, and step to the right. Throw your arms back over your head and reach behind you. Push your hips forward, keeping your feet parallel and your toes pointed forward.

Knees are straight

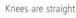

3 Exhale, step back with your feet together and bring your arms down. Stretch down to hold your ankles, pulling your forehead down to your knees.

Hips as high as possible

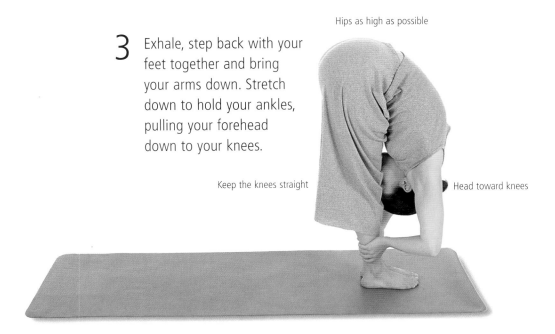

Keep the knees straight

Head toward knees

4 Place your palms down on the floor in preparation for the next move. If you cannot keep your legs straight, bend your knees slightly.

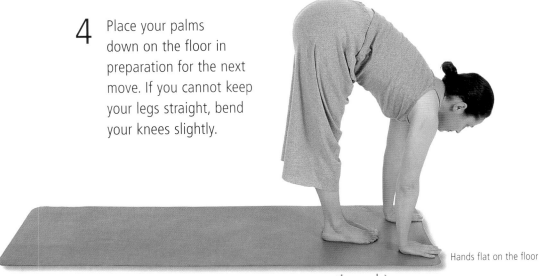

Hands flat on the floor

continued ▶

5 Inhale, and reach your right leg behind you. Balance on your toes, and bend your left knee. This is the position a sprinter adopts when preparing for a race.

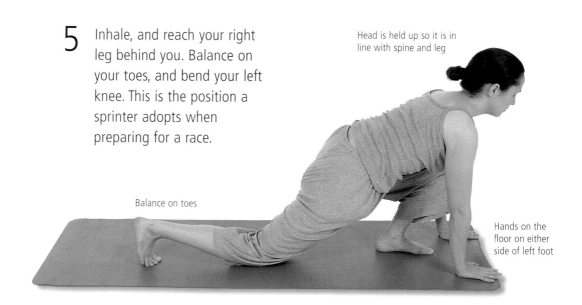

Head is held up so it is in line with spine and leg

Balance on toes

Hands on the floor on either side of left foot

6 Drop your right knee to the floor. Balance your weight at the top of your kneecap, but not on the kneecap itself, to prevent injury. Lift up your spine, raising your arms over your head with your palms together. Breathe normally and hold for a few seconds as you stretch.

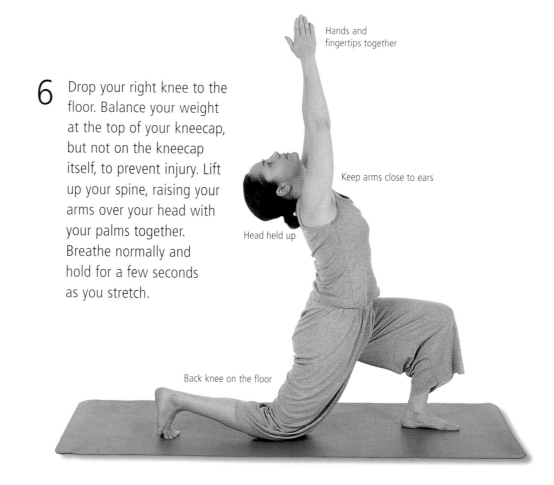

Hands and fingertips together

Keep arms close to ears

Head held up

Back knee on the floor

7 Release down to the position for Step 5, and drop your head with your chin toward your knee.

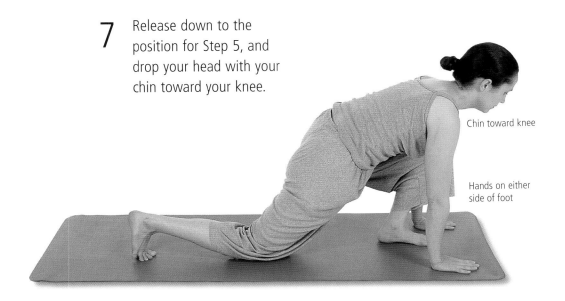

Chin toward knee

Hands on either side of foot

8 Leave your palms on the floor, inhale, and stretch out both legs behind you. Keep your elbows straight, and balance on your hands and feet. Keep your chin up and look forward.

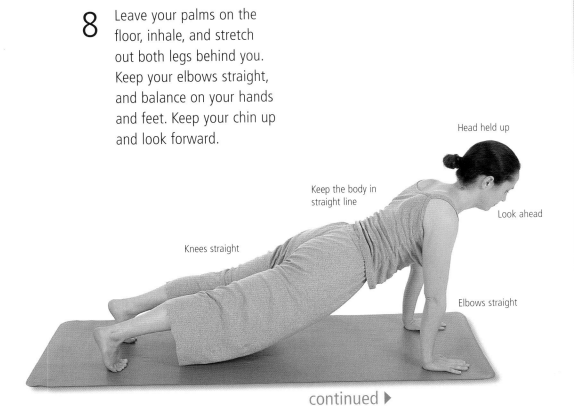

Head held up

Keep the body in straight line

Look ahead

Knees straight

Elbows straight

continued ▶

9 Exhale, drop both your knees to the floor, and look down to your hands.

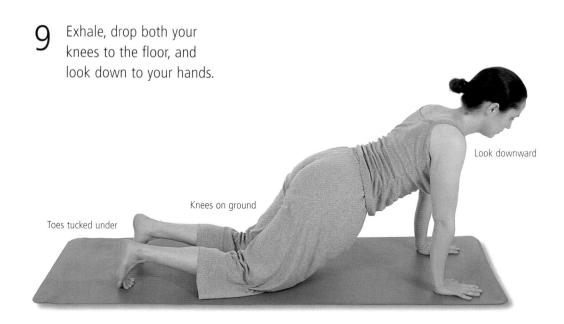

Look downward

Knees on ground

Toes tucked under

10 Continue to exhale and sit back on your heels, stretching out your arms in front of you to release your spine.

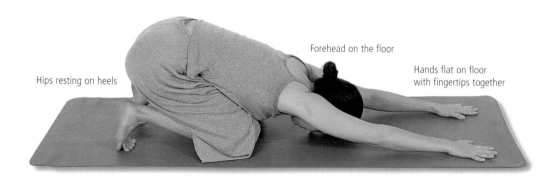

Forehead on the floor

Hands flat on floor with fingertips together

Hips resting on heels

11 Inhale again and dive forward like a snake, keeping your chin near the floor to make your spine flexible. Bend your elbows.

Hips upward

Bend elbows outward

Head straight in line to the floor

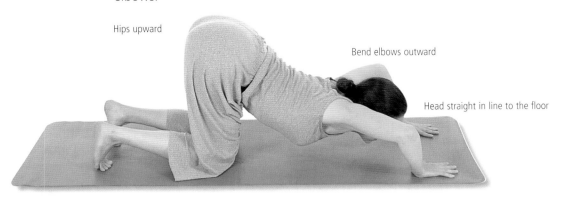

12 Continue inhaling, and move forward, sliding out your chest and chin so that they are close to the floor.

Hips upward

Chin toward floor

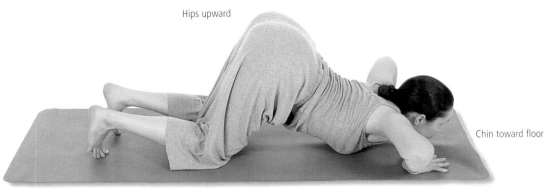

continued ▶

13 Still inhaling, drop your hips down and straighten your arms into the Cobra pose. Curve your spine, turning your head up. Exhale and return to Step 8, lifting your body up onto your toes again. Breathe normally.

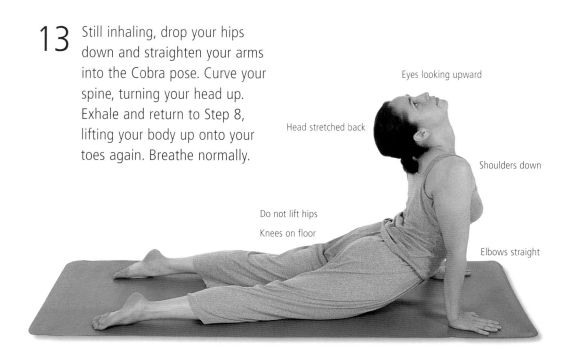

Eyes looking upward

Head stretched back

Shoulders down

Do not lift hips

Knees on floor

Elbows straight

14 Inhale, then as you exhale, raise your hips, extending your spine. Keep your heels down on the floor, and feel the stretch from your feet through your legs, spine, arms, and into your fingers. This position is the Dog pose. Breathe normally and hold for a few seconds.

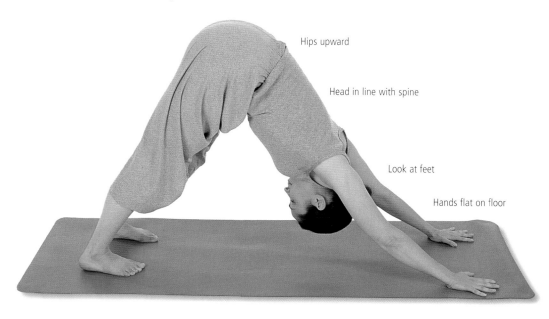

Hips upward

Head in line with spine

Look at feet

Hands flat on floor

15 Return to the Step 5 pose, but with your left leg back and your right knee bent with your right sole and palms flat on the floor. Look forward.

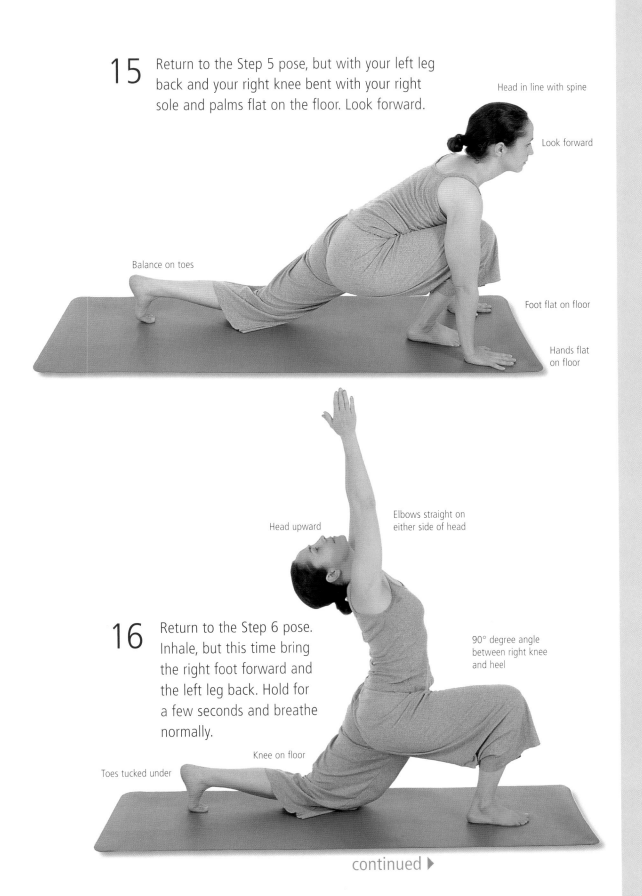

Head in line with spine

Look forward

Balance on toes

Foot flat on floor

Hands flat on floor

Head upward

Elbows straight on either side of head

16 Return to the Step 6 pose. Inhale, but this time bring the right foot forward and the left leg back. Hold for a few seconds and breathe normally.

90° degree angle between right knee and heel

Knee on floor

Toes tucked under

continued ▶

17 Exhale, stepping back with your feet together, and bring your arms forward to return to the Step 3 position.

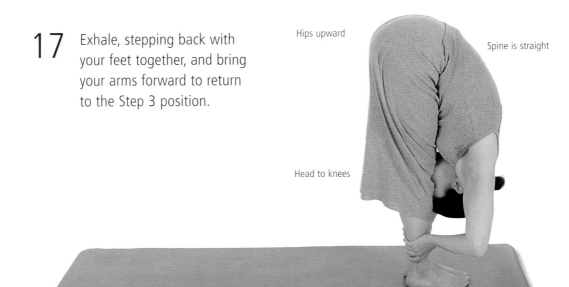

Hips upward

Spine is straight

Head to knees

Fingertips together with palms facing upward

Arms in line close to ears

Look upward

Arch the back

Hips forward

18 Inhale, and step to the left. Throw your arms out behind you and bend backward as far as possible, as in Step 2.

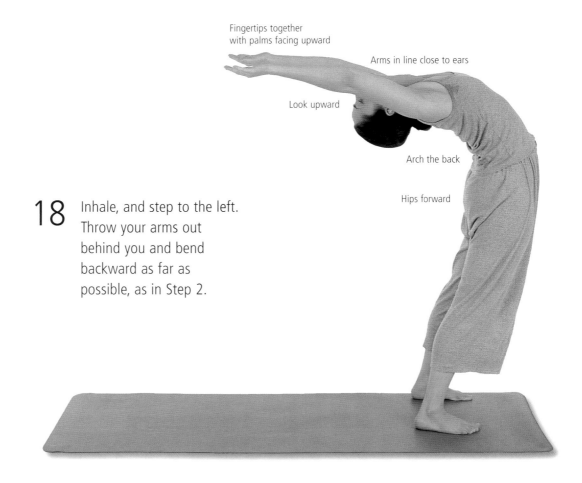

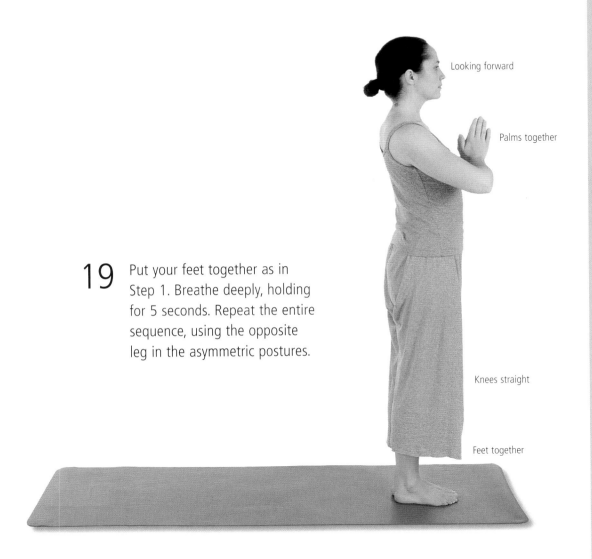

Looking forward

Palms together

19 Put your feet together as in Step 1. Breathe deeply, holding for 5 seconds. Repeat the entire sequence, using the opposite leg in the asymmetric postures.

Knees straight

Feet together

yoga for
exercise

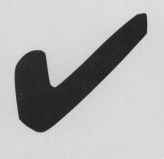

Many people don't realize that yoga exercise keeps you fit. The definition of fitness is "the ability to maintain normal physical activity without feeling fatigued." You don't need the strength and endurance of a marathon runner, but you should be able to perform your normal activities and have a reserve of energy.

The four types of fitness

There are 4 types of fitness to bolster health. The first is cardiorespiratory fitness. This refers to the fitness of your heart, lungs, and blood vessels. The better your cardiorespiratory fitness, the more stamina you have, and this lowers the risk of a host of diseases like heart disease, diabetes, and cancer.

The second is muscular fitness, which includes muscular strength and muscle endurance. Without exercise, all of us lose muscle mass as we age, which can result in weakness and loss of balance and coordination.

The third type of fitness is flexibility. As most people age, their muscles shorten and their tendons, the tissues that connect muscles to bones, become stiffer. This reduces the range of motion in the knees, shoulders, elbows, and other joints, as well as the spine. Loss of flexibility may be associated with an increased risk of pain and injuries.

The fourth fitness is body composition—the percentage of fat in your body. With the advancement of scientific testing, experts now agree that yoga improves fitness on all levels.

Why is yoga different?

Yoga exercise differs from other types of movement because of the emphasis on stretching and holding the postures. Stretching releases tension trapped in the muscles caused by stress, and, combined with yoga breathing techniques, tones and shapes the muscles while boosting energy levels. As you hold the pose, the energy has time to alter in the body, building strength and endurance. Jumping from movement to movement, as seen in aerobics or dance classes, merely depletes energy rather than builds energy levels.

Yoga gradually changes your physical body for the better. Not only will you see muscular definition, you will start to see a change in your habits toward moderation. You will cease to crave excesses and you will lose weight in a truly effective way. There will be no need for dieting, and you will return to the perfect you.

Warm-up

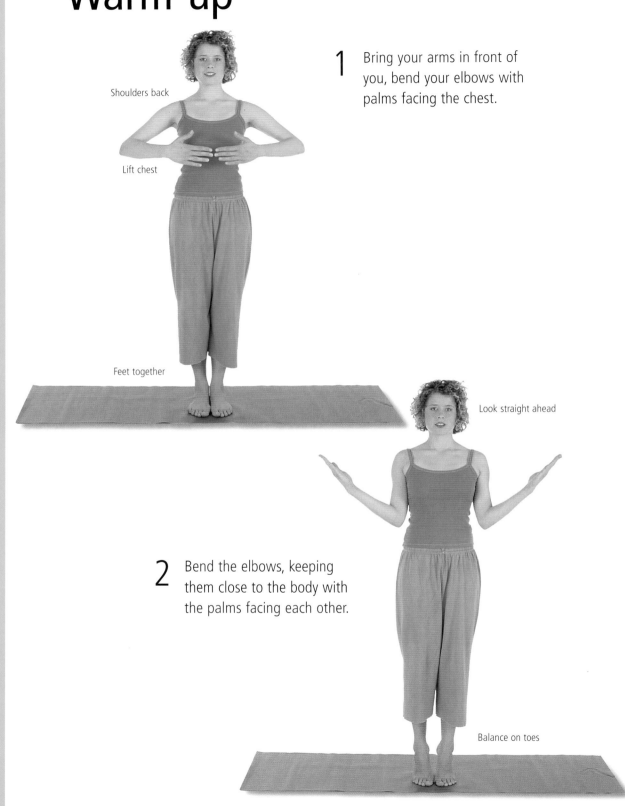

Shoulders back

Lift chest

Feet together

1 Bring your arms in front of you, bend your elbows with palms facing the chest.

Look straight ahead

2 Bend the elbows, keeping them close to the body with the palms facing each other.

Balance on toes

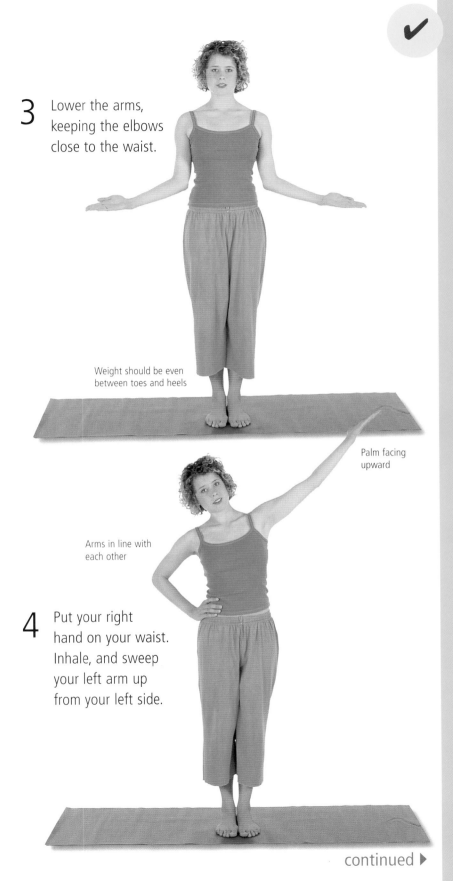

3 Lower the arms, keeping the elbows close to the waist.

Weight should be even between toes and heels

Palm facing upward

Arms in line with each other

4 Put your right hand on your waist. Inhale, and sweep your left arm up from your left side.

BENEFITS

This series of movements will gently warm up the muscles, which is necessary to avoid injury before starting any yoga postures. Before you begin, focus your attention on the breath and inhale and exhale through the nose in order to center the body and calm the mind. Stretching upward and to each side will loosen stiffness in the neck and shoulders and will allow energy to flow smoothly through the spine. You will feel energized, and as you move from one position to the next, try to be graceful like a dancer.

Physical
• Improves flexibility
• Increases energy levels

Mental
• Focuses the mind

Health
• Improves circulation

continued ▶

WARM-UP

43

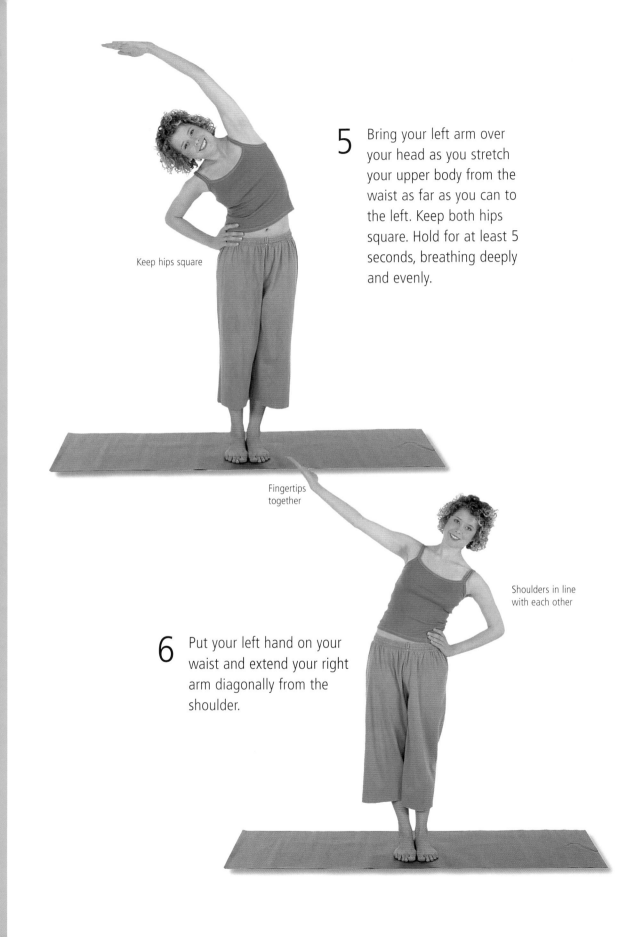

5 Bring your left arm over your head as you stretch your upper body from the waist as far as you can to the left. Keep both hips square. Hold for at least 5 seconds, breathing deeply and evenly.

Keep hips square

Fingertips together

Shoulders in line with each other

6 Put your left hand on your waist and extend your right arm diagonally from the shoulder.

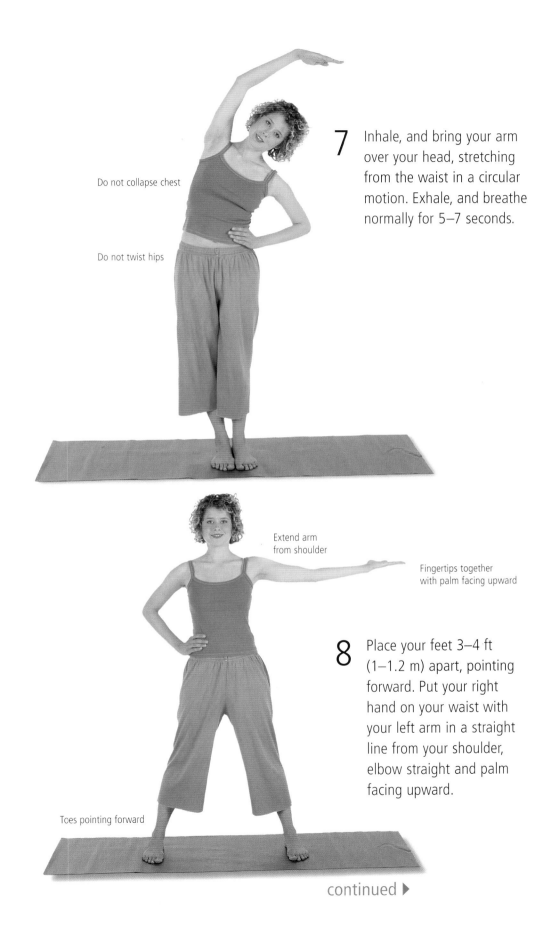

Do not collapse chest

Do not twist hips

7 Inhale, and bring your arm over your head, stretching from the waist in a circular motion. Exhale, and breathe normally for 5–7 seconds.

Extend arm from shoulder

Fingertips together with palm facing upward

8 Place your feet 3–4 ft (1–1.2 m) apart, pointing forward. Put your right hand on your waist with your left arm in a straight line from your shoulder, elbow straight and palm facing upward.

Toes pointing forward

continued ▶

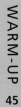

WARM-UP

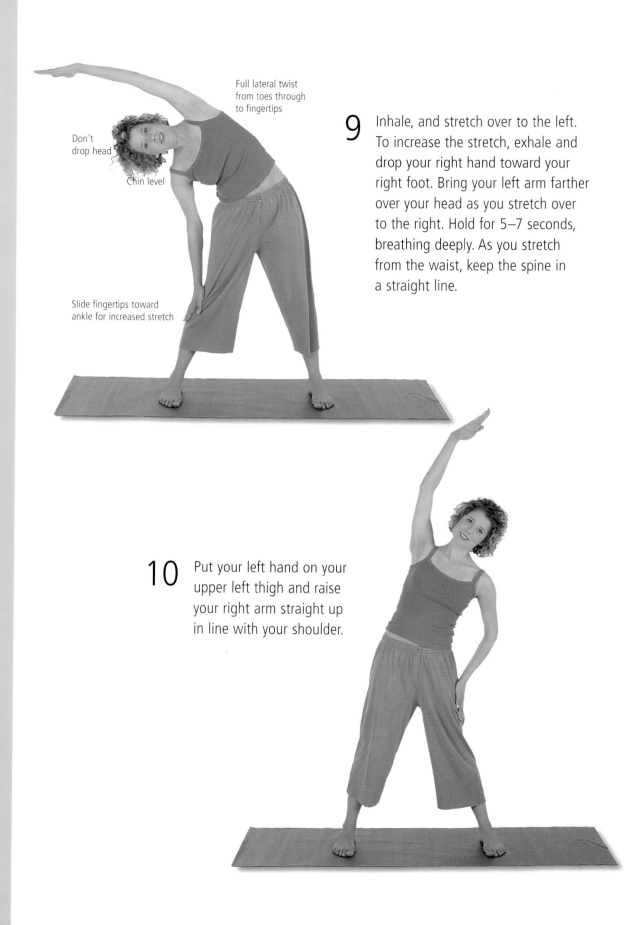

Full lateral twist
from toes through
to fingertips

Don't
drop head

Chin level

Slide fingertips toward
ankle for increased stretch

9 Inhale, and stretch over to the left. To increase the stretch, exhale and drop your right hand toward your right foot. Bring your left arm farther over your head as you stretch over to the right. Hold for 5–7 seconds, breathing deeply. As you stretch from the waist, keep the spine in a straight line.

10 Put your left hand on your upper left thigh and raise your right arm straight up in line with your shoulder.

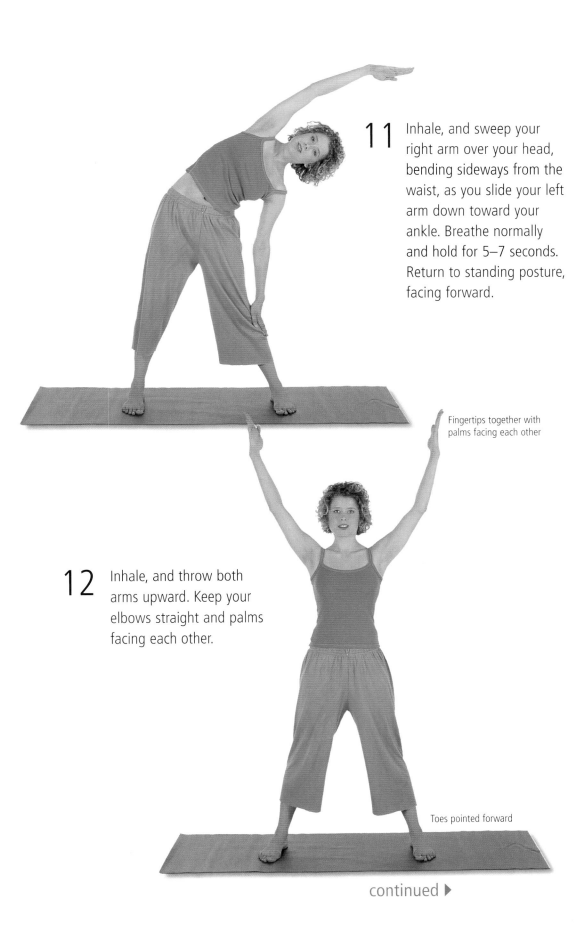

11 Inhale, and sweep your right arm over your head, bending sideways from the waist, as you slide your left arm down toward your ankle. Breathe normally and hold for 5–7 seconds. Return to standing posture, facing forward.

Fingertips together with palms facing each other

12 Inhale, and throw both arms upward. Keep your elbows straight and palms facing each other.

Toes pointed forward

continued ▶

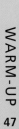

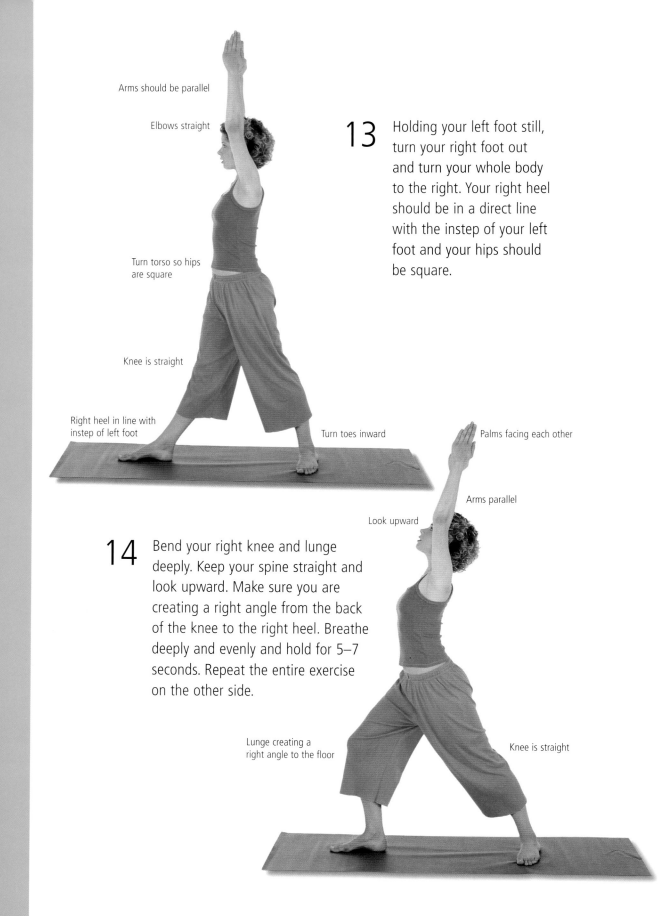

Arms should be parallel

Elbows straight

Turn torso so hips are square

Knee is straight

Right heel in line with instep of left foot

Turn toes inward

13 Holding your left foot still, turn your right foot out and turn your whole body to the right. Your right heel should be in a direct line with the instep of your left foot and your hips should be square.

Palms facing each other

Arms parallel

Look upward

14 Bend your right knee and lunge deeply. Keep your spine straight and look upward. Make sure you are creating a right angle from the back of the knee to the right heel. Breathe deeply and evenly and hold for 5–7 seconds. Repeat the entire exercise on the other side.

Lunge creating a right angle to the floor

Knee is straight

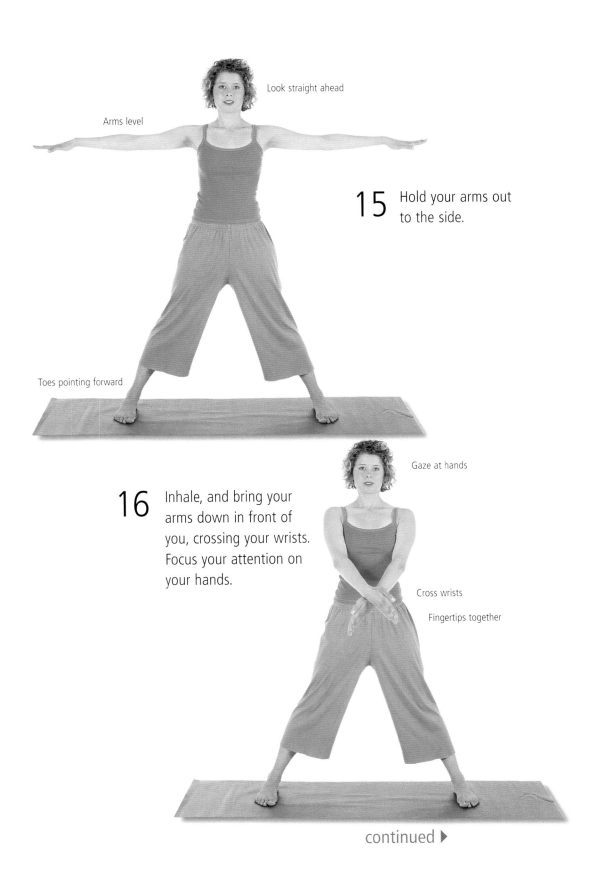

Look straight ahead

Arms level

15 Hold your arms out to the side.

Toes pointing forward

Gaze at hands

16 Inhale, and bring your arms down in front of you, crossing your wrists. Focus your attention on your hands.

Cross wrists

Fingertips together

continued ▶

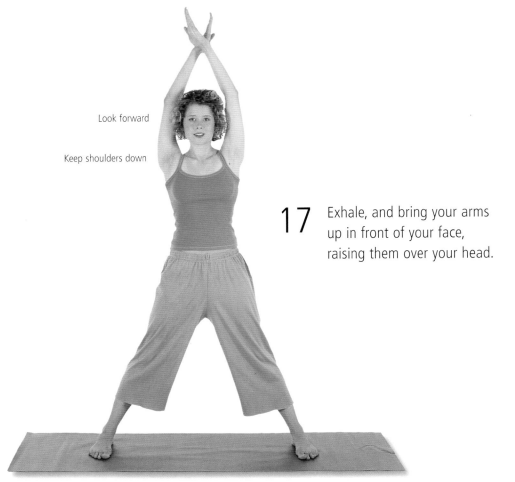

Look forward

Keep shoulders down

17 Exhale, and bring your arms up in front of your face, raising them over your head.

18 Inhale, and as you exhale, release both hands with a burst of energy. Leaving your arms up, inhale, and as you exhale, drop your body forward, bringing your arms down toward the floor.

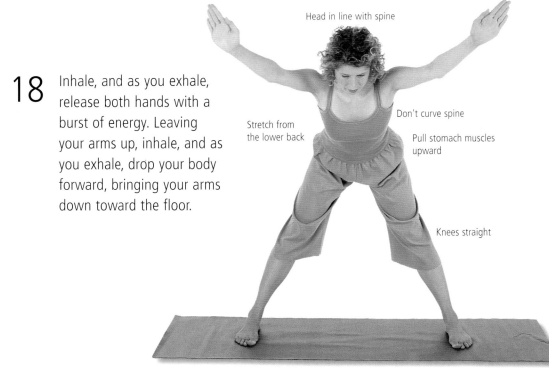

Head in line with spine

Don't curve spine

Stretch from the lower back

Pull stomach muscles upward

Knees straight

19 Breathe deeply and evenly and allow your natural body weight to take you down farther. If your spine is stiff and you are unable to lower yourself to the floor, do not force or jerk your body. You will be surprised at how fast your suppleness and flexibility will improve with this simple exercise. Hold for 5–7 seconds.

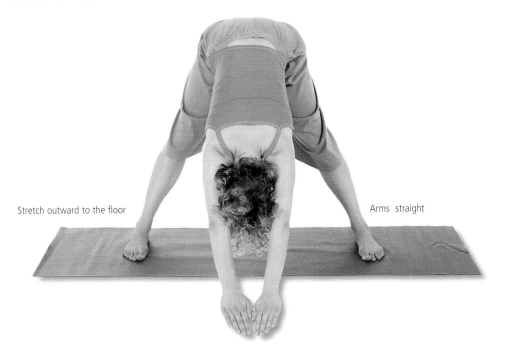

Stretch outward to the floor

Arms straight

20 Pull your tummy muscles up and stretch farther, holding your ankles and lowering your head toward the floor. Hold for 5 seconds, then slowly uncurl your spine and return to standing position.

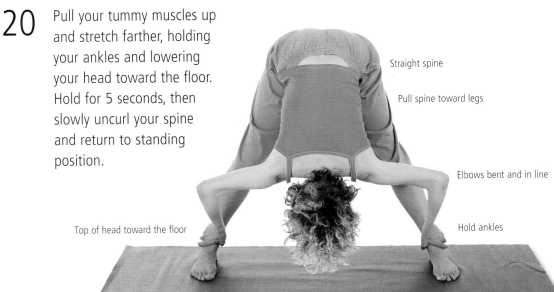

Straight spine

Pull spine toward legs

Elbows bent and in line

Top of head toward the floor

Hold ankles

Triangle

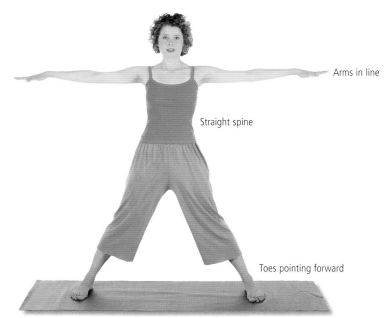

Arms in line

Straight spine

Toes pointing forward

1 Stand up straight and place your feet about 3 ft (1 m) apart. Stretch out your arms with your palms facing down. Keep them in line with your shoulders. Breathe normally.

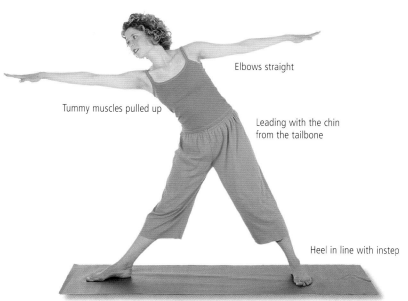

Elbows straight

Tummy muscles pulled up

Leading with the chin from the tailbone

Heel in line with instep

2 Turn in your left foot slightly and point your right foot 90° to the right. Inhale and stretch to the right. Keep the spine straight and do not tilt forward. Breathe normally, and hold for 5 seconds.

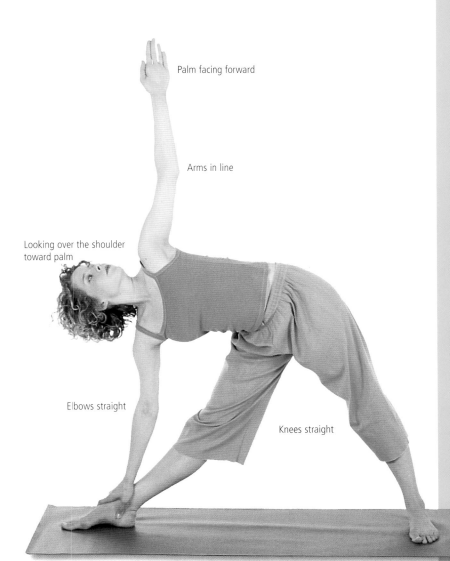

Palm facing forward

Arms in line

Looking over the shoulder toward palm

Elbows straight

Knees straight

BENEFITS

This is a total lateral stretch, which improves muscle tone, especially in the ankles, legs, hips, and arms. It also revitalizes the spinal nerves and abdominal organs. As you stretch to the side, think of stretching from the tailbone. There is a tendency to collapse the spine and twist either forward or backward. The triangle looks very simple, but the alignment of the body is very precise. The angles of the spine, arms, and legs are very important.

Physical
- Increases flexibility of hips, spine, and legs
- Stretches spine

Mental
- Helps anxiety
- Reduces mental stress

Health
- Improves circulation
- Helps constipation and stomach disorders
- Helps cure sciatica and lower back pain

Ayurvedic
- Good for all types, especially *Vata*

3 Place your right hand on your right ankle, and extend your left arm up in a straight line with your palm facing forward. Look up toward your arm, keeping your head up. Relax your face and shoulders, and hold for 10 seconds.

Warrior 1

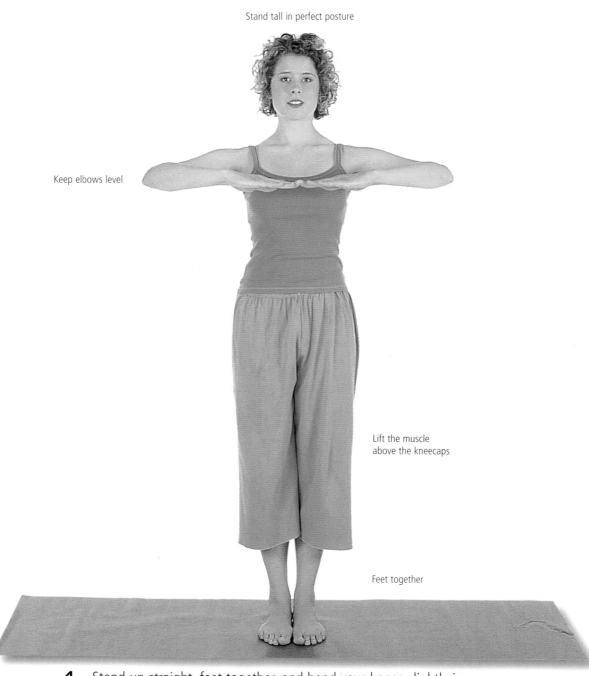

Stand tall in perfect posture

Keep elbows level

Lift the muscle
above the kneecaps

Feet together

1 Stand up straight, feet together, and bend your knees slightly in
preparation to jump. Bring your arms up to shoulder level, and
place your fingertips together.

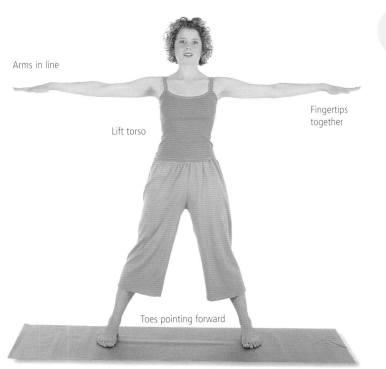

Arms in line

Lift torso

Fingertips together

Toes pointing forward

2 Jump to open your legs wide—they should be about 4 ft (1.2 m) apart. Make sure your toes are pointing forward and stretch both your arms out sideways.

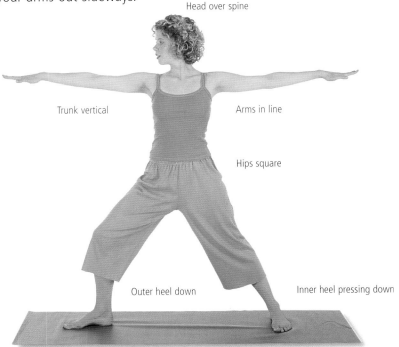

Head over spine

Trunk vertical

Arms in line

Hips square

Outer heel down

Inner heel pressing down

3 Turn your right knee and face to the right. Lean your body backward, and push your hips and stomach forward. Now bend your right knee, keeping your spine straight. Bend farther until there is a 90° angle between your thigh and the floor. Repeat on the other side.

BENEFITS

The Warrior is a powerful and dynamic standing pose that empowers the mind and body. Although it is a static pose, it is meant to be held for at least 30 seconds; it is only then that you will feel invigorated and energized. You will feel your breath deepen as you hold the pose, as vital *prana* is pushed throughout the entire system, nourishing and revitalizing all cells.

Physical
- Strengthens legs
- Trims thighs

Mental
- Creates positive mental attitude
- Increases awareness and sensitivity

Health
- Rejuvenates cells through increased oxygen in blood

Warrior 2

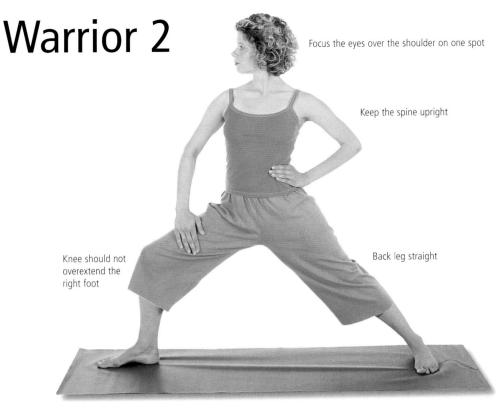

Focus the eyes over the shoulder on one spot

Keep the spine upright

Back leg straight

Knee should not overextend the right foot

1 Stand with your feet 3–4 ft (1–1.2 m) apart, arms to the side. Turn your right foot to the right with your right heel in a direct line to the instep of your left foot. Bend your right knee in a 90° angle so the back of the knee is in line with the right heel. Place your right hand on your inner thigh and your left hand on your waist. Breathing normally, hold for 5–7 seconds.

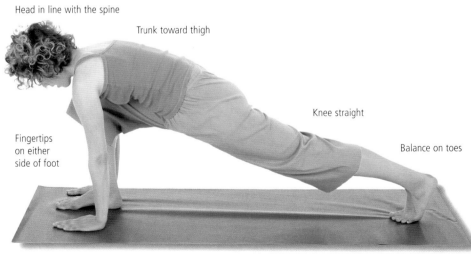

Head in line with the spine

Trunk toward thigh

Knee straight

Fingertips on either side of foot

Balance on toes

2 Turn your body to the right, and place your fingertips on the floor. Turn your left foot so it is in line with your right heel.

BENEFITS

This extended twist increases suppleness and flexibility of the spine as well as develops strength and stamina. It is a difficult pose and needs practice to gain balance and poise. Make sure you can do the first Warrior pose before attempting this. The twist massages and stimulates the internal organs helping digestive disorders.

Physical
- Increases suppleness of spine
- Increases flexibility
- Improves balance
- Improves strength and stamina
- Trims stomach

Mental
- Challenges mind
- Aids concentration

Health
- Massages internal organs
- Invigorates liver, kidney, spleen, and colon

Ayurvedic
- Good for *Vata* and *Kapha* types

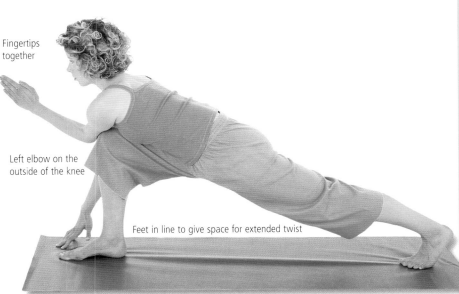

Fingertips together

Left elbow on the outside of the knee

Feet in line to give space for extended twist

3 Bend your left arm, and place your elbow on the outside of your right knee. Keep your fingers together and look down at your palm.

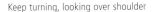

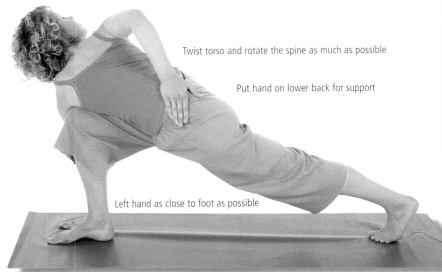

Keep turning, looking over shoulder

Twist torso and rotate the spine as much as possible

Put hand on lower back for support

Left hand as close to foot as possible

4 Inhale, twist your spine to the right and look over your right shoulder. Reach your right hand around to your left hip and put your left hand on the floor beside your right leg. Exhale, breathe deeply and hold for 7–10 seconds. Release, stand tall and repeat on the other side.

WARRIOR 2

Back bend

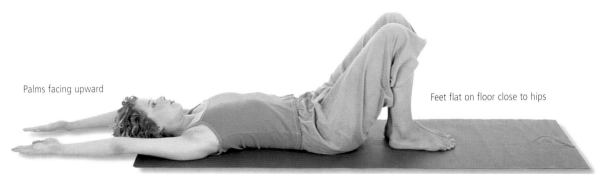

Palms facing upward

Feet flat on floor close to hips

1 Lie flat on the floor, and bring your knees up. Place your feet as close to your body as possible. Stretch both your arms out behind your head, and breathe normally.

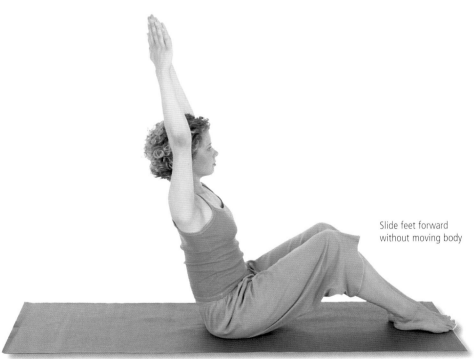

Slide feet forward without moving body

2 Inhale and sit up tall, stretching your arms upward in line with the side of your head. Stretch out your legs slightly, but keep your feet together. Breathe normally.

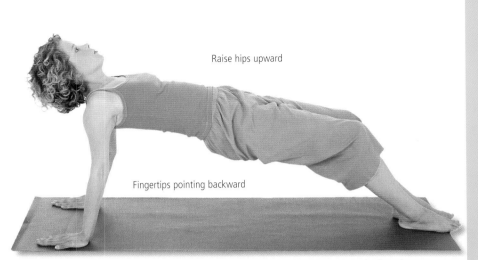

Raise hips upward

Fingertips pointing backward

3 Keeping your feet flat on the floor, balance your arms behind you. Point your palms away from your feet to support your body weight. Inhale and lift your buttocks, keeping an even line between your knees, hips, and shoulders. Look up, exhale, and breathe normally for 5 seconds.

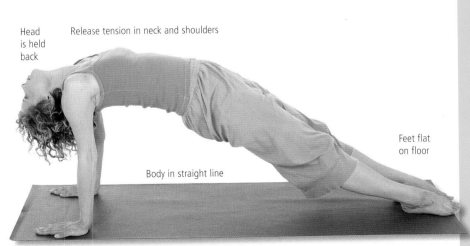

Head is held back

Release tension in neck and shoulders

Feet flat on floor

Body in straight line

4 Inhale, extend your legs and straighten your knees. Drop your head back and relax the neck and face. Keep pushing your hips upward. Breathing normally, hold for 5 seconds.

BENEFITS

Back bends stimulate and energize the spine. This exercise also releases the fear of going backward. In yoga practice, we bend forward, sideways, and backward to balance the total flexibility of the body. It strengthens the shoulders, arms, and hips, as well as develops coordination and stamina. It is important to feel that it is releasing any tension in the spine, so make sure your face and jaw are both relaxed.

Physical
- Strengthens arms, shoulders, and wrist
- Increases flexibility and mobility of hips
- Improves stamina

Mental
- Improves mental endurance
- Improves mental concentration

Health
- Keeps one youthful
- Prevents backache
- Helps arthritis

Ayurvedic
- Good for *Kapha* types

Leg lift

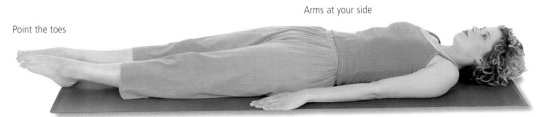

Point the toes   Arms at your side

1 Lie flat on the floor with your arms at your sides. Keep your eyes open and gaze up, breathing deeply and slowly.

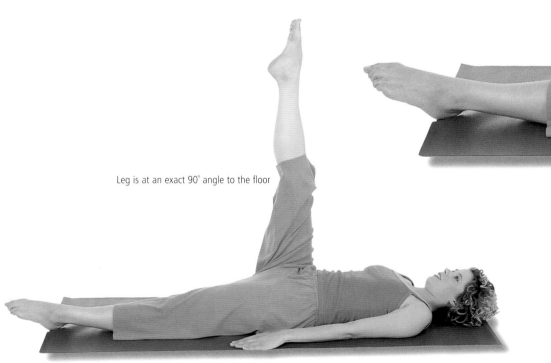

Leg is at an exact 90° angle to the floor

2 Inhale, and raise your right leg at a 90° angle to the other leg. Hold still for 5 seconds, breathing normally.

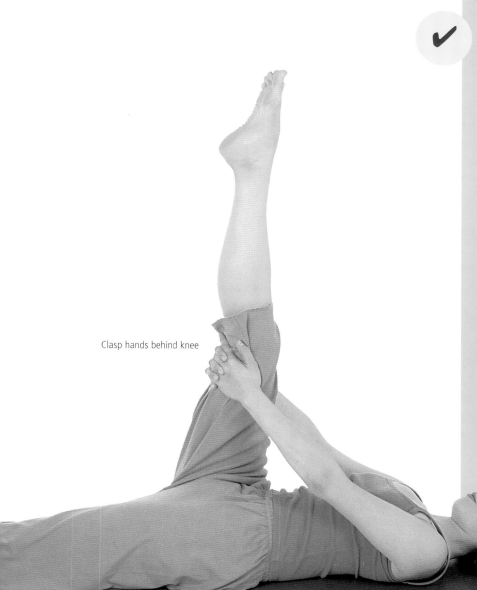

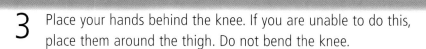
Clasp hands behind knee

BENEFITS

This exercise strengthens the abdominal muscles and increases the flexibility of the hips and hamstrings. Concentrate on the breathing as you move from one position to the next. In the beginning you might find it difficult to stretch your leg to your head. As you practice you will feel your stomach muscles working as you raise both legs and head off the floor.

Physical
- Flattens stomach
- Increases suppleness of spine
- Stretches hamstrings

Mental
- Focuses mind
- Improves mental coordination

Ayurvedic
- Good for *Pitta* types

3 Place your hands behind the knee. If you are unable to do this, place them around the thigh. Do not bend the knee.

continued ▶

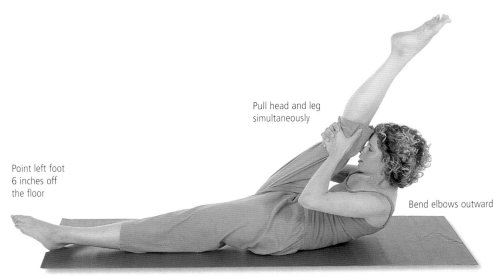

Pull head and leg
simultaneously

Point left foot
6 inches off
the floor

Bend elbows outward

4 Bring your forehead up to your knee and hold for 5 seconds. Point your left foot about 6 in (15 cm) off the floor.

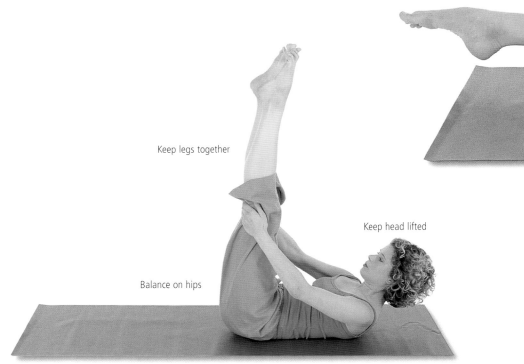

Keep legs together

Keep head lifted

Balance on hips

5 Bring both feet together, pointing your toes up. As you hold as still as possible for 5 seconds, you will feel your stomach muscles at work.

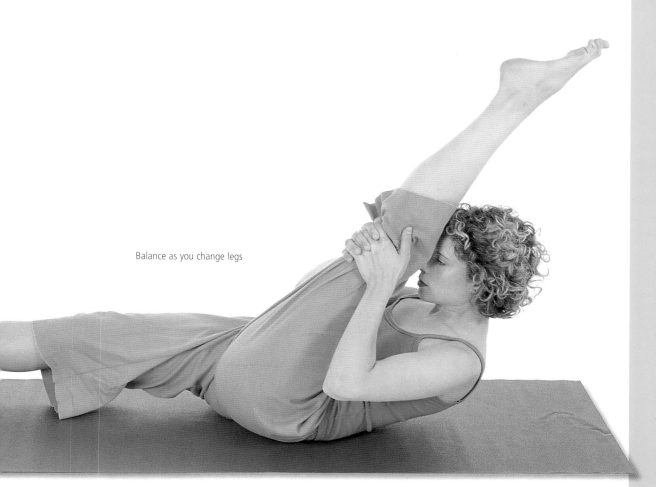

Balance as you change legs

6 Bring your left leg and forehead together and lower the right leg to 6 in (15 cm) off the floor. Repeat steps 4–6 several times.

Sitting balance

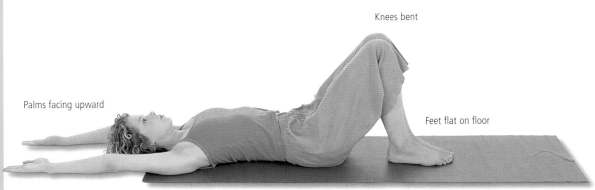

Knees bent

Palms facing upward

Feet flat on floor

1 Lie flat on your back with your knees up and your feet together on the floor. Take your arms back over your head.

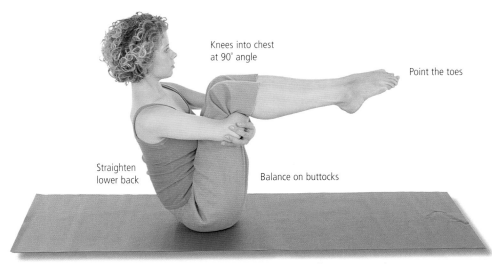

Knees into chest at 90° angle

Point the toes

Straighten lower back

Balance on buttocks

2 Inhale and stretch up, pulling the knees into your chest. Straighten your spine and balance on your buttocks. Breathe normally.

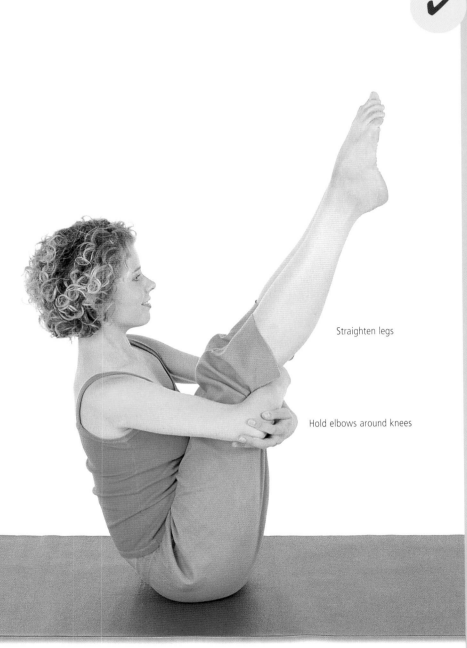

Straighten legs

Hold elbows around knees

3 Straighten your knees and point your toes. Do not collapse the spine. Hold your stomach in for 10–15 seconds.

continued ▶

BENEFITS

This exercise combines balance with a full forward stretch of the spine. It also strengthens the lower back. Remember that both the abdominal and back muscles are working to keep the balance. As you stretch the legs and torso forward, stretch from the chest rather than the head. Breathing evenly and deeply throughout the exercise will increase stamina and flexibility.

Physical
- Flattens stomach
- Stretches hips, spine, and muscles at the back of legs
- Massages abdominal organs
- Increases flexibility of the spine
- Improves coordination and balance

Mental
- Improves concentration
- Increases mental endurance
- Enhances visualization

Health
- Tones digestive organs
- Cures nervous disorders
- Relieves constipation
- Regulates pancreatic function
- Helps sciatica and back problems in lumbar region

Ayurvedic
- Excellent and beneficial to all *doshas*

SITTING BALANCE

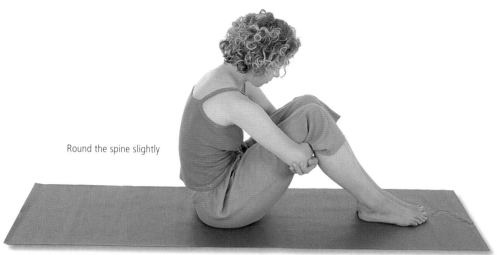

Round the spine slightly

4 Exhale and relax forward, bringing your feet down to the floor.
Bend your head slightly, and curve the spine.

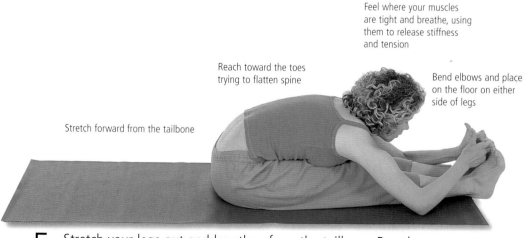

Feel where your muscles
are tight and breathe, using
them to release stiffness
and tension

Reach toward the toes
trying to flatten spine

Bend elbows and place
on the floor on either
side of legs

Stretch forward from the tailbone

5 Stretch your legs out and lengthen from the tailbone. Breathe
normally, extending your chin forward. Put your fingers around
your big toes and flex the thumbs.

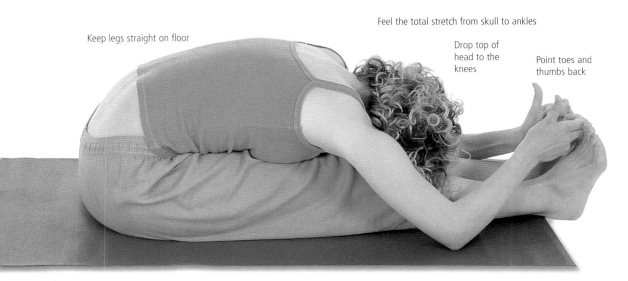

Keep legs straight on floor

Feel the total stretch from skull to ankles

Drop top of head to the knees

Point toes and thumbs back

6 Extend forward as far as you can, then drop your forehead to your knees for 20 seconds. To release, sit tall and relax back.

One-arm balance

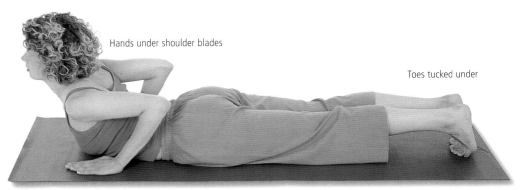

Hands under shoulder blades

Toes tucked under

1 Lie flat on to the floor. Tuck your toes under and keep the legs straight. Place your hands directly under the shoulder blades and bend the elbows. Look straight ahead.

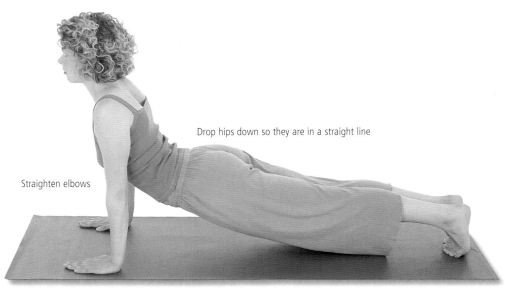

Drop hips down so they are in a straight line

Straighten elbows

2 Inhale, push the palms down to the floor and lift your entire body off the floor. Keep the hips down. Tighten the stomach muscles and buttocks, and stretch the legs fully. Exhale, breathe normally, and hold for 10 counts.

BENEFITS

This is a challenging exercise that requires strength, stamina, flexibility, and balance. This also helps boost energy levels with the principle that the more energy you use, the more energy you have. The shoulders, upper arms, and forearms are especially strengthened as you push up into the position. When you keep your feet, legs, hips, torso, and head in a straight line your weight on either side will be perfectly balanced.

Physical
- Strengthens arms
- Increases energy levels
- Improves stamina

Mental
- Increases mental endurance
- Improves concentration
- Challenges mind

Health
- Builds immune system

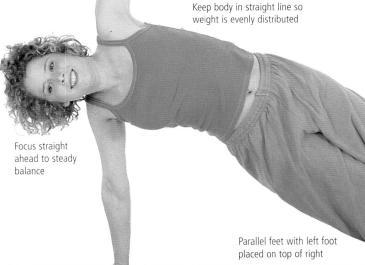

Palm facing forward

Keep body in straight line so weight is evenly distributed

Focus straight ahead to steady balance

Parallel feet with left foot placed on top of right

3 Inhale deeply, swing the body to the right, balancing on the right hand. Stretch the left arm up. Make sure that your feet are parallel and your body is in a straight line so that you can balance on one arm. Exhale, then inhale deeply, and hold for 5–10 counts.

Ayurvedic
- *Vata* types enjoy this exercise and *Pitta* and *Kapha* need it to build muscular strength

continued ▶

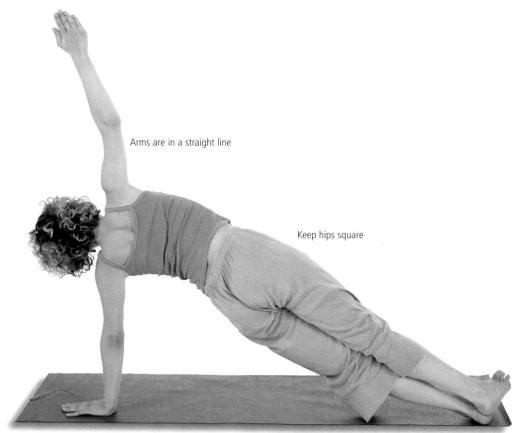

Arms are in a straight line

Keep hips square

4   Inhale, swing to the other side so you are balancing on your left hand. Exhale, breathe deeply. Make sure you are in a straight line and your right arm is in line.

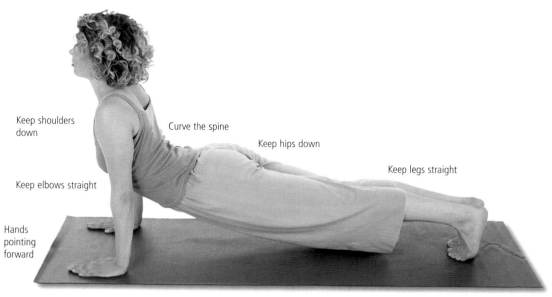

Keep shoulders down

Curve the spine

Keep hips down

Keep legs straight

Keep elbows straight

Hands pointing forward

5   Swing back to the center, and balance between your toes and hands. Keep your body a few inches off the floor to strengthen the arms.

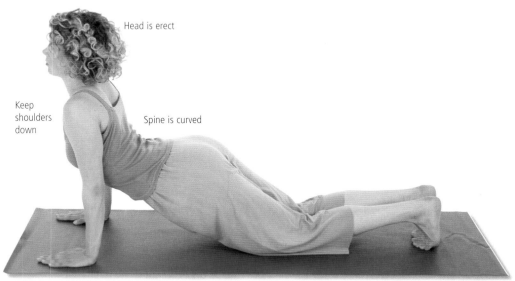

Head is erect

Keep shoulders down

Spine is curved

6 Slowly drop to the knees, keeping the spine curved upward.

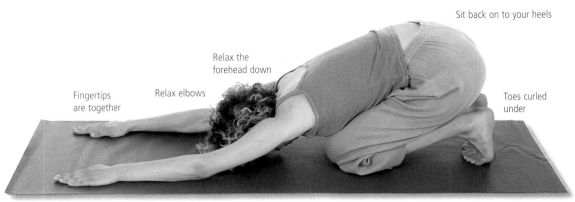

Sit back on to your heels

Relax the forehead down

Fingertips are together

Relax elbows

Toes curled under

7 Keeping your hands in the same place, stretch your hips back toward your heels and sit back on your ankles. Drop your forehead down to the floor. Inhale and exhale. Relax in the position for at least 10–15 counts.

Letter T

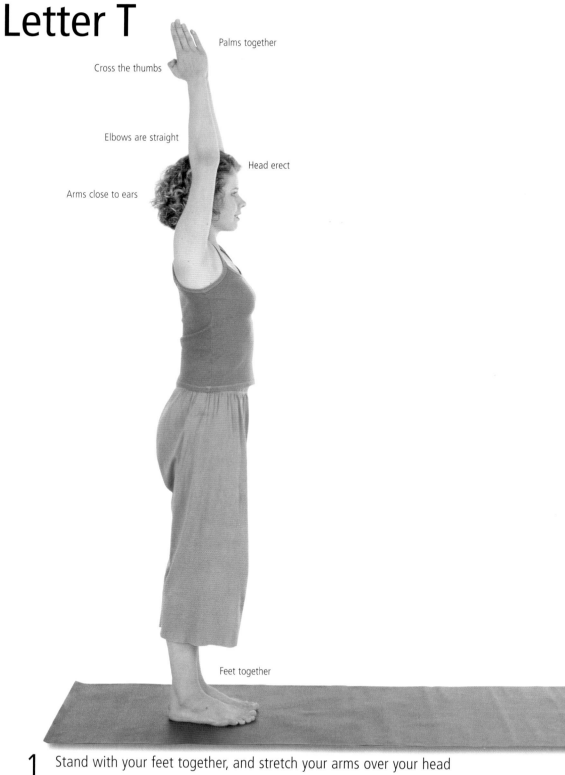

Palms together

Cross the thumbs

Elbows are straight

Head erect

Arms close to ears

Feet together

1 Stand with your feet together, and stretch your arms over your head
close to the ears. Bring your palms together and cross your thumbs.
Keep the elbows straight. Keep your shoulders down and spine
straight. Inhale and exhale, and focus your eyes straight ahead.

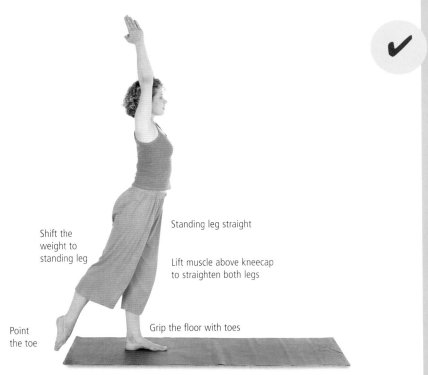

Shift the weight to standing leg

Standing leg straight

Lift muscle above kneecap to straighten both legs

Point the toe

Grip the floor with toes

2 Shift the weight to the left leg, point your right foot, and extend the right leg behind you slightly off the floor. Keep both knees straight. Focus on one spot ahead of you.

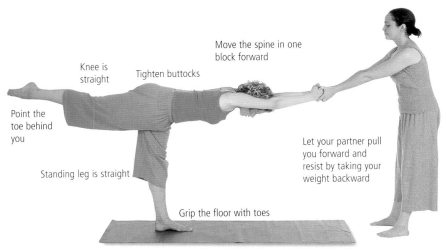

Move the spine in one block forward

Knee is straight

Tighten buttocks

Point the toe behind you

Standing leg is straight

Let your partner pull you forward and resist by taking your weight backward

Grip the floor with toes

3 In one movement, stretch forward keeping the spine straight, and simultaneously take the right leg up behind you so you look like the letter T. Keep the hips square, and stretch from the tailbone in either direction. Your partner should stand in front of you, hold your hands, and help you stretch forward. As he or she pulls you gently forward, keep stretching backward to straighten the spine so it is flat. Distribute the weight evenly between the arms and legs. Your breath will quicken, so breathe deeply and evenly from the diaphragm while holding the pose for 10–15 counts.

BENEFITS

This posture is a difficult exercise for beginners, but when you master the pose, you will enjoy the many benefits. This is the only yoga pose that is held for no longer than 10 seconds. The position of the arms over the head raises the pulse rate and the breath quickens. This is a cardiovascular exercise that burns calories and increases oxygen levels. As the breath quickens, deepen the inhalation in order to get the maximum results.

Physical
- Increases stamina
- Raises energy levels
- Tones buttocks and upper arms

Mental
- Improves balance
- Enhances focus and concentration
- Increases willpower

Health
- Improves circulation
- Strengthens lungs
- Helps prevent heart disease

Ayurvedic
- Excellent for *Vata* types

Jet

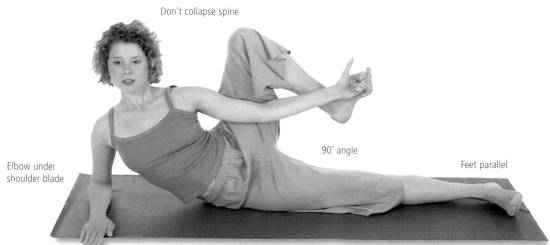

Don't collapse spine

90° angle

Elbow under
shoulder blade

Feet parallel

1 Lie balanced on your elbow, making sure it is under your shoulder blade. Flex both feet and keep your knees straight. Bend the left knee and take hold of the big toe with your thumb flexed. Your left thigh should be at a 90° angle to the right leg.

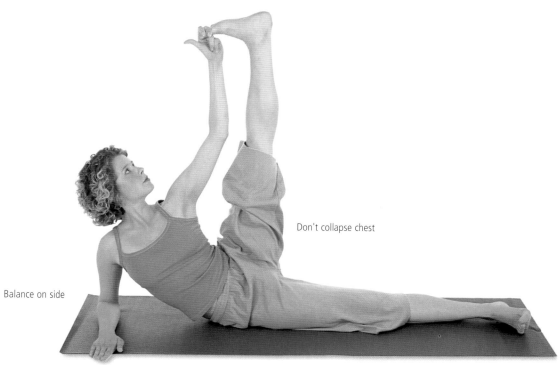

Don't collapse chest

Balance on side

2 Inhale and straighten your left leg, making a 90° angle with the right leg. Flex the toes.

BENEFITS

This is a fast-paced exercise that improves circulation and increases overall flexibility and stamina. It also tones abdominal muscles, buttocks, and legs. Try to flow from one movement to the next without jerking. In the final position hold for as long as possible to allow the energy to alter in the body.

Physical
- Flattens stomach muscles
- Tones buttocks muscles
- Stretches neck muscles

Mental
- Calms the mind
- Improves mental balance

Health
- Calms nervous system
- Massages internal organs
- Helps digestive disorders

Ayurvedic
- Good for *Vata* types

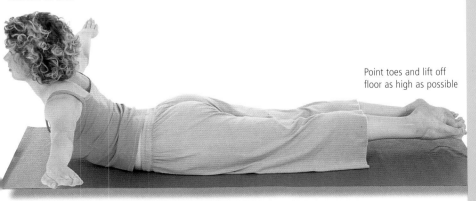

Lift chin off floor

Point toes and lift off floor as high as possible

3 Exhale, release your foot and swing over onto your stomach. Raise head and limbs off the floor.

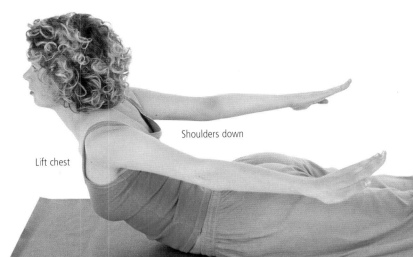

Lift chin upward to stretch neck

Shoulders down

Lift chest

4 Inhale, raising your arms behind to lift your chest. Hold for 10 seconds, breathing normally. Exhale, and relax for 20 seconds.

Spinal twist 1

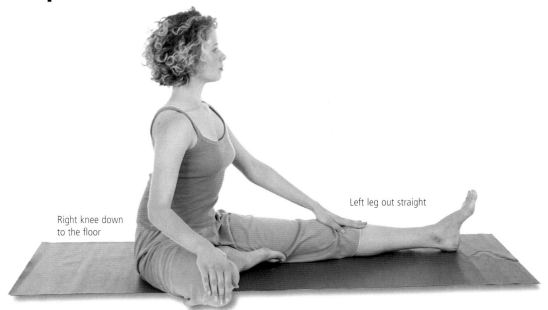

Right knee down
to the floor

Left leg out straight

1 Sit on the floor with both legs stretched straight out in front of you. Flex your right foot and take your right leg into a half lotus. Sit upright and try to bring your right knee down to the floor. Breathe normally.

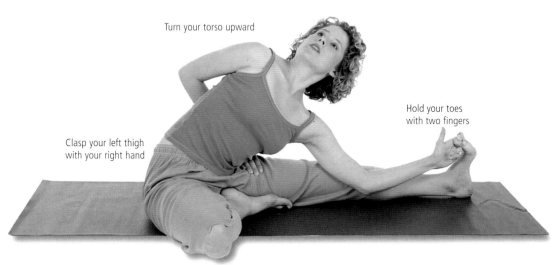

Turn your torso upward

Hold your toes
with two fingers

Clasp your left thigh
with your right hand

2 Reach sideways toward your left foot, bend your elbow and clasp two fingers around the foot, extending your thumb. Twist your spine and look over your right shoulder. Take your right arm around the lower back and hold your left thigh. Keep twisting and turn your torso upward. Breathe deeply and hold for 10 seconds.

BENEFITS

All twists are very effective in relieving backaches. As the torso turns, the kidneys and abdominal organs are activated. This action helps remove harmful toxins that build up in the internal organs over time. Digestion is improved and digestive disorders are often cured. The turning of the hips makes the spine more supple giving more mobility in the hip joint.

Physical
- Opens the hip
- Increases mobility of the spine
- Increases flexibility

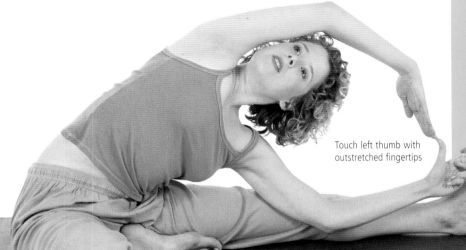

Touch left thumb with outstretched fingertips

3 Release your right arm and bring it sideways over your head to touch the left thumb. Keep your head even between your arms. Breathing normally, hold for 10 seconds. Repeat on the other side.

Mental
- Soothes nerves

Health
- Cures digestive disorders
- Aids digestion process
- Releases toxin build-up
- Relieves headaches
- Relieves backache
- Tones abdominal organs, kidneys, and spleen

Ayurvedic
- Good for *Kapha* types

Breathe & relax 1

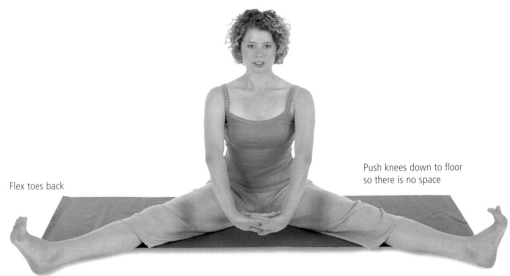

Flex toes back

Push knees down to floor so there is no space

1 Sit on the floor with your legs wide apart. Flex your toes upward and try to push your knees down to the floor. Clasp your fingertips together in front of you.

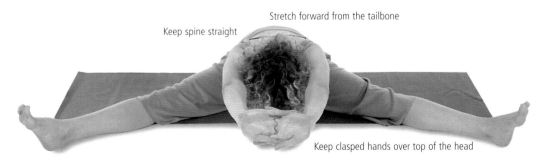

Keep spine straight

Stretch forward from the tailbone

Keep clasped hands over top of the head

2 Inhale, lean forward and stretch your arms out, keeping your hands up over your head. Turn your thighs outward to increase the stretch.

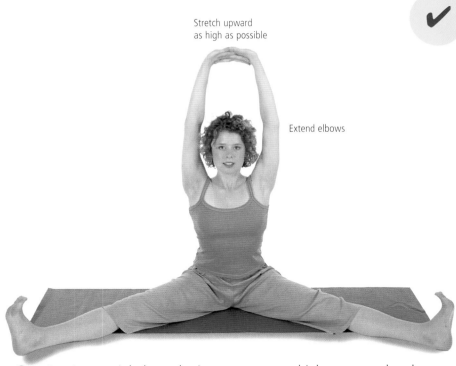

Stretch upward as high as possible

Extend elbows

3 Continue to inhale, and raise your arms up high over your head. Sit as tall as you can and open your chest, keeping your shoulders down.

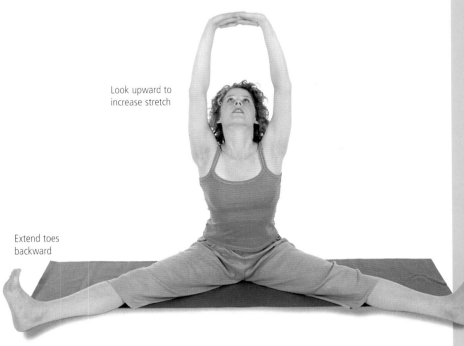

Look upward to increase stretch

Extend toes backward

4 Exhale, drop your head back, and look up to your clasped palms. Do not cave in at the chest or release your lower back. Inhale again and return to Step 3.

continued ▶

BENEFITS

Stretching to your maximum is an ideal way to release tension in the muscle groups. When you combine it with deep breathing, the mind becomes calm and the brain relaxed. As you breathe deeply through these movements, your flexibility will improve. Don't worry if you cannot manage the last position when your head is down on the floor. With continued practice with an understanding of the importance of breath, you will see a marked difference in your flexibility.

Physical
- Improves flexibility
- Increases suppleness of the spine
- Opens the hips

Mental
- Relieves stress
- Calms and soothes the nervous system

Health
- Increases oxygen in the blood supply
- Rejuvenates all cells in the body

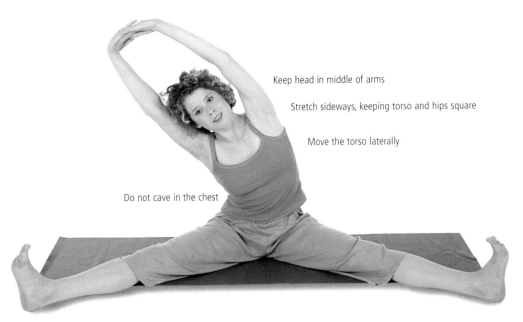

Keep head in middle of arms

Stretch sideways, keeping torso and hips square

Move the torso laterally

Do not cave in the chest

5 Stretch sideways from the waist, keeping the torso and hips square. Keep the head in the middle of the arms. Keep the knees straight and flex the toes. Inhale and exhale and hold for 5 counts.

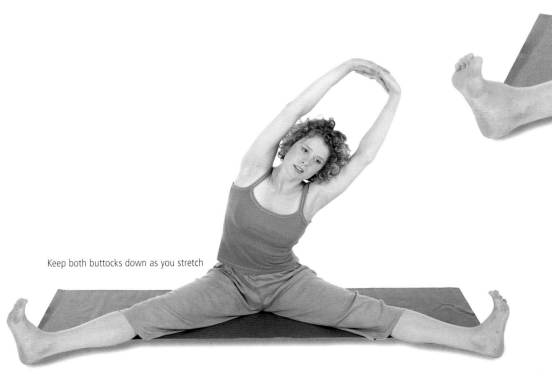

Keep both buttocks down as you stretch

6 Repeat on the other side. Make sure to keep buttock muscles down to the floor. Inhale, exhale, and hold for 5 counts.

Breathe and relax slowly down into the pose

Never jerk or force your body

Don't force head down

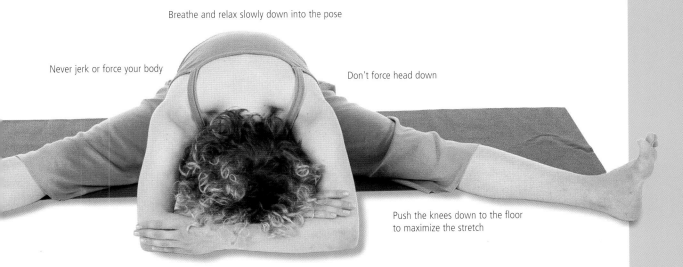

Push the knees down to the floor
to maximize the stretch

7 Slowly lower the body forward so your forehead reaches the floor. Never
force your body and head down. Breathe deeper and deeper and slowly
relax in the position. Cross your elbows over your head. Inhale and
exhale deeply and hold for 15–20 counts.

FACE & THROAT

As we age, the muscles in the face and neck tend to sag. Like the rest of the muscles in the body, they need to be stretched to stay taut and youthful. Increased oxygen in the cells will replenish and rejuvenate the cells. This improves the appearance of wrinkles and helps to improve the complexion and sagging jowls. Yoga exercise improves circulation because of the twisting, turning, and inverted positions of the body.

Fish

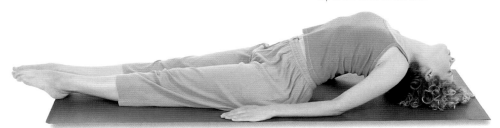

Arch your back upward and rest top of the head on the floor

1 Lie on the floor with your arms out and point your toes. Inhale and raise your chest, resting your weight on the crown of your head. Feel the stretch in your neck and face. Exhale and breathe normally, holding for 3 seconds.

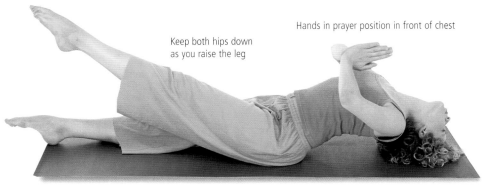

Keep both hips down as you raise the leg

Hands in prayer position in front of chest

2 Still balancing on your head, inhale and raise your left leg, keeping your hip on the floor. Place your palms together above your chest, holding for 3 seconds. As you exhale, lower your leg slowly. Relax to the floor, if necessary, before Step 3.

This exercise focuses on the parathyroid glands, which are located in the throat. The position of the top of the head also stimulates and tones the pineal and pituitary glands. This position also expands the lungs fully which revitalizes the cervical, thoracic, and lumbar regions of the spine. It also improves circulation to the face and slows the aging process. The stiffness of the neck and shoulders are released and respiratory problems are alleviated.

Physical
- Clears complexion
- Promotes sparkling eyes
- Releases tension in neck and shoulders
- Tones abdominal muscles
- Corrects rounded shoulders

Mental
- Regulates mood swings
- Relieves stress

Health
- Helps cure respiratory ailments like asthma and bronchitis
- Increases lung capacity

Ayurvedic
- Good for all *doshas*

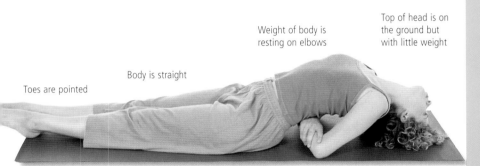

Do not strain face and neck

Top of head is on the ground but with little weight

Weight of body is resting on elbows

Body is straight

Toes are pointed

3 Place your arms under your lower back, clasping your elbows. Keep raising your chest upward and continue to point your toes.

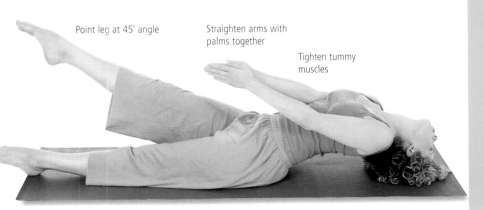

Point leg at 45° angle

Straighten arms with palms together

Tighten tummy muscles

4 Inhale and raise your right leg, raising your chest. Extend your arms up with your palms together. Hold for 5 seconds. Exhale, lower your right leg, then release the neck and chest down slowly, relaxing to the floor. Hold for 10 seconds. Repeat on the other side.

NECK & SHOULDERS

When people are stressed, the muscles in the neck and shoulders tighten, and in severe cases, seize up. It is important to have a simple and effective way to release this tension. Yoga exercise eases the muscles, and deep breathing calms and soothes the brain.

Shoulder release

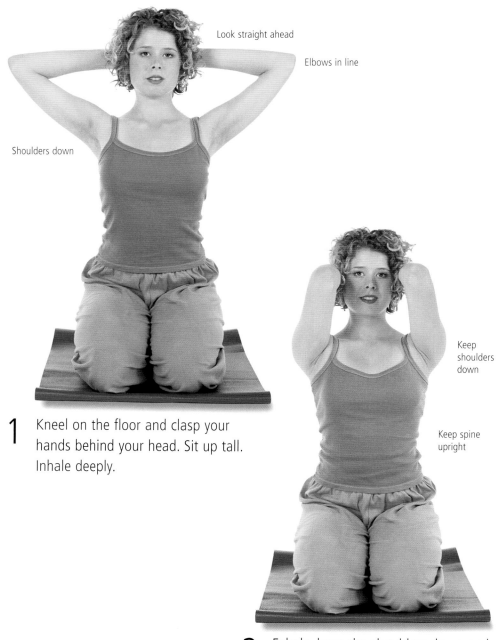

Look straight ahead

Elbows in line

Shoulders down

Keep shoulders down

Keep spine upright

1 Kneel on the floor and clasp your hands behind your head. Sit up tall. Inhale deeply.

2 Exhale, keep the shoulders down and bring the elbows toward each other.

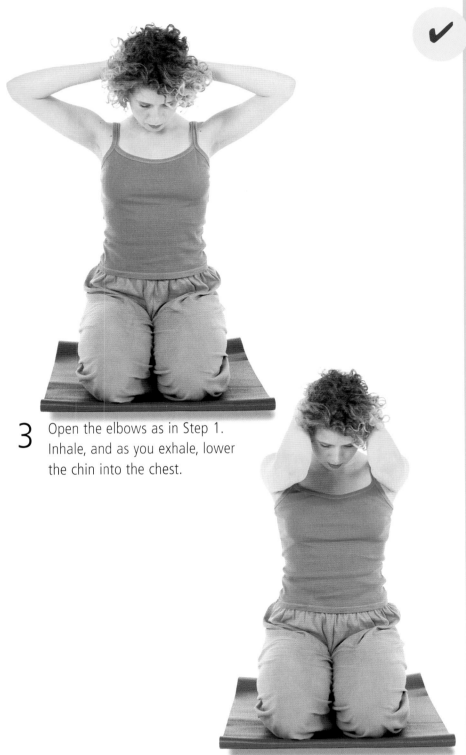

3 Open the elbows as in Step 1. Inhale, and as you exhale, lower the chin into the chest.

4 Inhale, and as you exhale, bring the elbows toward each other while keeping the chin locked into the chest. Inhale, and return to Step 1. Repeat the sequence 5 times.

BENEFITS

This exercise releases tension and stress in the neck, shoulders, and upper back. It also helps to relieve fatigue while acting as a natural tranquillizer for the nervous system. When you are calm and relaxed, emotional imbalances are reduced and you can face the stresses of modern living with clarity.

Physical
- Improves posture
- Relaxes face

Mental
- Calms the mind
- Provides clarity of thought
- Brings positive outlook
- Provides sunny disposition

Health
- Prevents stress disorders
- Restores harmony and balance
- Cures breathing disorders
- Regulates thyroid
- Balances metabolism

UPPER ARMS

It seems that the upper arms are the first to become flabby, even when the rest of the physical body is toned and supple. With sedentary living, we never have a real chance to use our arms so the muscles become weak. It is important to target this area with specific exercises that build strength and give definition and shape to the upper arms.

Push-ups

Palms and elbows on the floor

Forehead down toward the floor

Tuck the toes under

Fingertips together

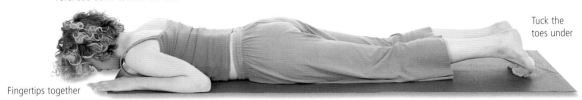

1 Lie flat on the floor with your face down. Tuck the toes under. Place your palms on the floor at either side of the head. Keep the elbows close to the body. Raise your head a few inches off the floor.

Curve the spine

Elbows in toward the body

Elbows are bent

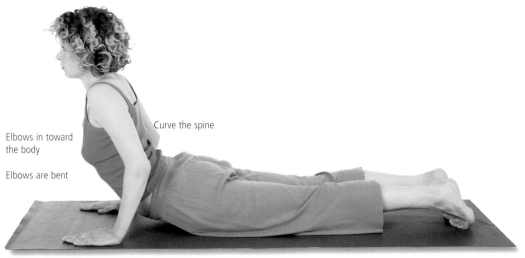

2 Inhale, push the palms down and curve your spine upward into a beautiful arch. Keep the elbows in toward the body. Exhale, breathe normally, and hold for 5 counts.

BENEFITS

This exercise will tone the upper arms, legs, and tummy. The final pose requires extra stamina, so build up your strength slowly.

Physical
- Builds physical strength
- Builds stamina
- Shapes and tones the arms
- Increases energy levels

Mental
- Boosts confidence
- Improves positive thinking
- Promotes strength of character

Health
- Builds immune system
- Releases stress
- Fights lethargy and fatigue

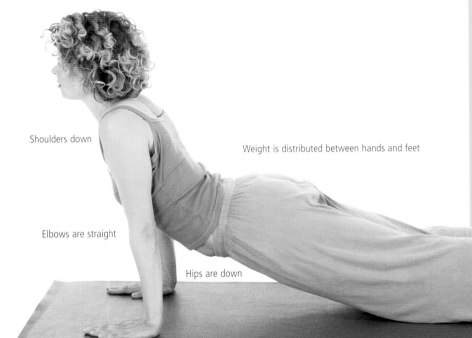

Shoulders down

Weight is distributed between hands and feet

Elbows are straight

Hips are down

3 Straighten the elbows. Lift the entire body off the floor while keeping the hips down. Inhale and exhale and hold for 5–10 counts. Lower the body down to Step 1. Relax for a few counts and repeat the sequence 3–5 times.

CHEST

The heart *chakra* rules emotions and sentiments, and when people are upset, they tend to cave the chest inward. Opening the chest boosts self-confidence. As you begin the back bends, the muscles should be soft and the mind mentally alert to the action. There should be no stress or strain in the movement. Push the shoulder blades down while lifting the chest upward, as this lifts the spine and head, giving a regal and powerful impression.

Camel

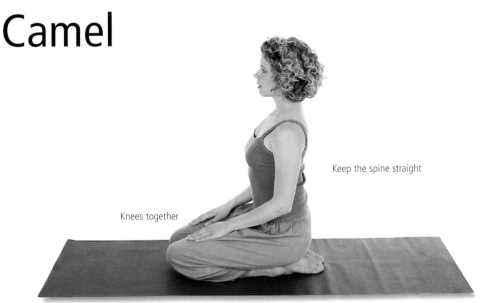

Keep the spine straight

Knees together

1 Kneeling on the floor, sit up tall with your arms resting on the thighs. Focus straight ahead. Inhale and exhale normally.

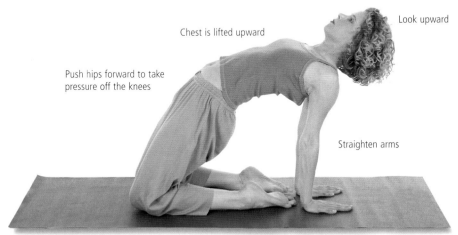

Chest is lifted upward

Look upward

Push hips forward to take pressure off the knees

Straighten arms

2 Bring the knees under the hip bones, inhale, and lift your hips and head upward. Shift your weight so the tops of the thighs and hips face upward. Exhale, arch the back, and place the hands on the floor behind you, close to the heels, with the fingertips facing the same direction as the feet. Breathe normally, and hold for 5 counts.

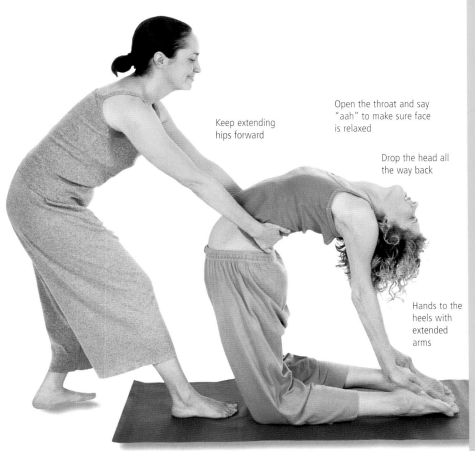

Keep extending hips forward

Open the throat and say "aah" to make sure face is relaxed

Drop the head all the way back

Hands to the heels with extended arms

3 Keep pushing the hips forward to create a beautiful arch in the spine. Open the chest and drop the shoulders. Turn the arms outward and hold on to the heels. Keep the thighs vertical, and drop the head back. Do not strain the face and neck. The throat should be open so you can say "aah." Breathe normally. Your partner should stand in front of you and pull you forward from the small of the back. This forces you to intensify the stretch and supports the lower back.

BENEFITS

This is an intense back stretch that rejuvenates the spine and releases all the muscular tension from the lower back to the top of the head. It also relaxes and soothes the nervous system. The chest is entirely open, which allows the lungs to expand to their full capacity. It is important to open the throat and relax the face, especially the jaw. Keep pushing the hips forward to achieve the maximum stretch. There should not be any weight in the legs. They should only act as an anchor for the full stretch.

Physical
- Builds muscles in the lower back
- Increases circulation to face and neck
- Has anti-aging effects
- Releases stress in the back, shoulders, neck, and face
- Strengthens thighs

Mental
- Relaxes the brain
- Soothes nervous system
- Calms the mind

Health
- Boosts immune system
- Relieves backache

ABDOMEN

The abdominal muscles represent the core muscles in the body. They need to be strong to lift your spine in perfect posture. People with weak muscles experience back pain and suffer from ailments such as lumbago and sciatica. In perfect posture, the muscles of the abdomen and lower back are working equally. Be aware of both muscle groups: Isolate the muscles, and tighten and release them to invigorate and tone the internal organs.

Stomach stretches

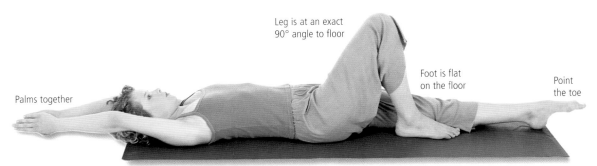

Leg is at an exact 90° angle to floor

Foot is flat on the floor

Point the toe

Palms together

1 Lie flat on the floor with your arms to the side. Bring your right knee up and place your right foot flat on the floor. Point your left foot and take both arms over your head. Place your palms together and straighten your elbows.

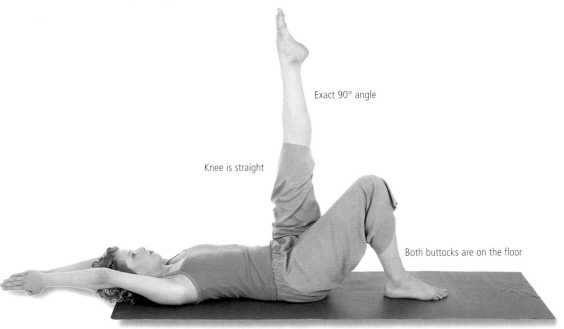

Exact 90° angle

Knee is straight

Both buttocks are on the floor

2 Inhale, keeping your left leg at a 90° angle to the floor. Exhale, breathe normally and hold for 5 seconds.

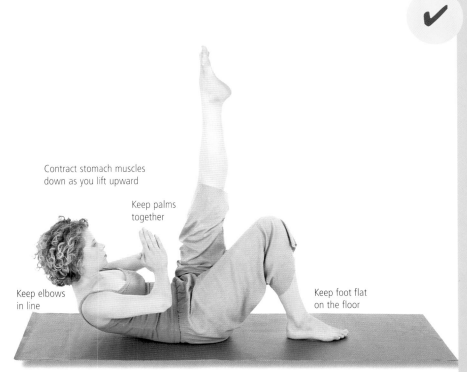

Contract stomach muscles
down as you lift upward

Keep palms
together

Keep elbows
in line

Keep foot flat
on the floor

3 Inhale and bring your palms in toward your head. Exhale, sit up,
and bring your arms down in front of your face above the chest.

Stretch arms

Keep elbows straight

Hold stomach muscles tight

4 Inhale, straighten your arms, exhale, breathe normally and hold for
5 seconds. Inhale, slowly lower your back, and bring your arms over
your head. Exhale, and then repeat the exercise on the other side.

BENEFITS

This series of movements
will tone the stomach
muscles and flatten the
stomach. Pay special
attention to the breathing
pattern, as incorrect usage
can produce the opposite
results. Always exhale as
you contract the tummy
muscles. Think of drawing
the muscles down toward
the floor while you are
tightening the stomach
muscles.

Physical
• Tones abdominal muscles
• Flattens stomach

Mental
• Improves concentration
• Promotes mental
  well-being

Health
• Prevents digestive
  disorders

ABDOMEN: STOMACH STRETCHES

WAIST

Stretching to the side helps to strengthen your abdominals and tone your waist, improving your body's flexibility and releasing tension in your lower back. Most people never bend or stretch sideways, unless they go to an exercise class, but as the body ages, it is very important to stay supple and maintain mobility. As you stretch sideways, keep your hips square and facing forward, and keep your feet firmly on the floor. Do not collapse your waist, but lengthen the spine from the hip as you extend right down to the floor.

Side stretch 1

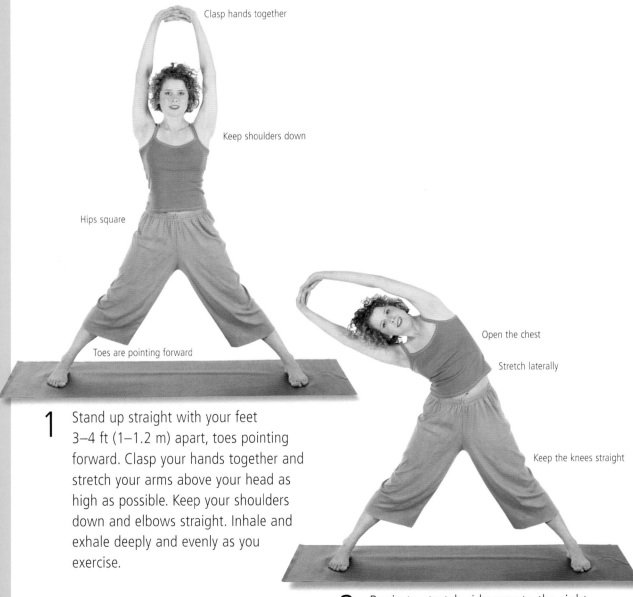

Clasp hands together

Keep shoulders down

Hips square

Toes are pointing forward

Open the chest

Stretch laterally

Keep the knees straight

1 Stand up straight with your feet 3–4 ft (1–1.2 m) apart, toes pointing forward. Clasp your hands together and stretch your arms above your head as high as possible. Keep your shoulders down and elbows straight. Inhale and exhale deeply and evenly as you exercise.

2 Begin to stretch sideways to the right from the waist.

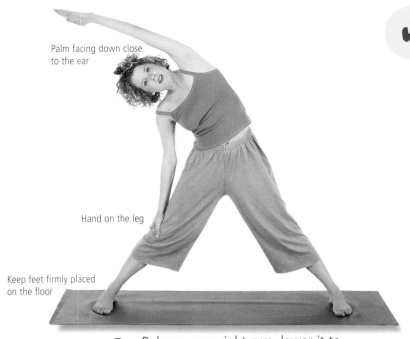

Palm facing down close to the ear

Hand on the leg

Keep feet firmly placed on the floor

3 Release your right arm, lower it to your knee and hold this position for a few seconds.

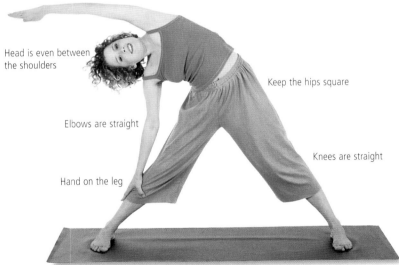

Head is even between the shoulders

Keep the hips square

Elbows are straight

Knees are straight

Hand on the leg

4 Move your right hand down toward your right ankle and hold for 10 seconds. As you improve your flexibility and increase your stretch, you will be able to reach all the way down with your palm onto the floor, keeping your arm and hips in a straight line. Release the stretch, stand up straight, and then repeat the exercise on the other side.

BENEFITS

Stretching to the side increases mobility of the spine while trimming your waistline. In yoga, we stretch in all directions in order to increase flexibility and release tension in the muscle groups. When stretching sideways, it is important not to collapse the chest. Hips tend to twist as you stretch. Think of the precision of the pose, not how far you can stretch. Don't force the body to go beyond its limit.

Physical
- Trims the waist
- Increases flexibility and mobility of the spine

Mental
- Maintains youthfulness
- Has a feel-good factor

Health
- Improves circulation
- Increases blood supply to the heart

BUTTOCKS

All yoga exercise strengthens and tones the buttock muscles. Yoga is total action, so every cell is active, vibrant, and full of life. Every movement, whether you are lifting, turning, extending, or pressing, involves the buttock muscles. Be aware of every muscle from your toes to your fingertips, and feel all the muscles working together in a complex interplay. If one part of the body is not sensitive or active, the pose is not complete.

Locust

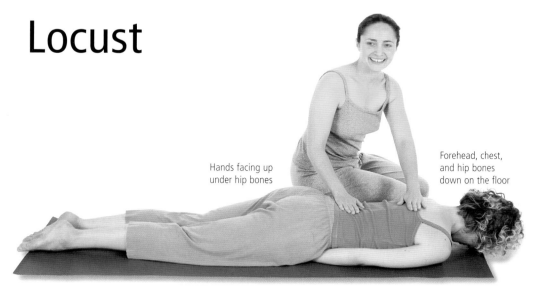

Hands facing up under hip bones

Forehead, chest, and hip bones down on the floor

1 Lie on the floor face down. Keep your back straight and hold your arms by your sides, with your hands under your thighs, with the palms up.

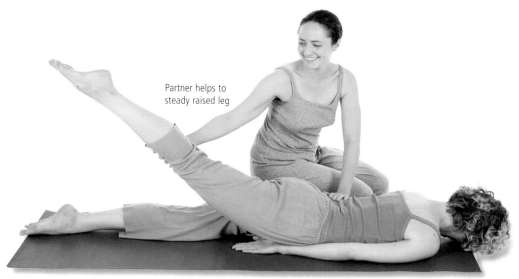

Partner helps to steady raised leg

2 Inhale and raise your right leg, keeping your hips square. Allow your partner to steady the leg, but not to support it. Breathe normally and hold for 6 seconds. On the last exhalation, slowly lower the leg, then inhale and repeat on the other side.

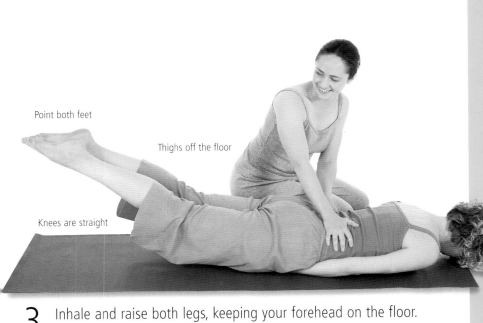

Point both feet

Thighs off the floor

Knees are straight

3 Inhale and raise both legs, keeping your forehead on the floor. Keep lifting, breathing deeply, for as long as you can. On the last exhalation, lower both legs. Repeat, then turn your head to one side and relax.

BENEFITS

The Locust tightens and tones the buttock muscles, flattens the tummy and strengthens the legs. When you lift the leg upward, keep the hip bones down on the floor. This forces you to tighten the buttocks before you begin to lift the leg, and as you hold the pose, the buttock muscles are isolated and strengthened. Do not worry if you cannot lift the legs very high. Think of extending out from the hip bone rather than raising the leg. It is a challenging exercise that builds endurance and stamina, but with continued practice you will find it less strenuous.

Physical
- Tones legs and buttocks
- Increases energy levels
- Helps flatten stomach

Mental
- Increases mental endurance
- Increases willpower
- Improves concentration

Health
- Stimulates digestive organs
- Massages internal organs
- Aids digestion
- Relieves gastric troubles and flatulence
- Stimulates prostate gland in men
- Strengthens bladder and ovaries in women

yoga for
health

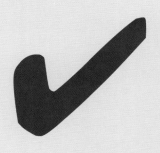

The most important aim of our lives should be to maintain good health. Many people take their health for granted and abuse their bodies with a sedentary lifestyle, bad diets, medications, and high stress factors. In order to prevent disease, we must make a conscious decision to combat the ills of modern living and improve our attitude toward health. Every person, due to genetic weaknesses, is susceptible to certain ailments that if not prevented can lead to serious illnesses. When energy is depleted in the body, the organs become weak and they cannot function properly. The natural equilibrium will be disturbed and a disorder can develop. Genetic factors will dictate which particular disorder may develop and which organ might be affected. Some people may be prone to a certain condition such as diabetes, cancer, peptic ulcers, or heart disease.

How Ayurvedic practice can help

The Indian medical philosophy known as *Ayurvedic* medicine believes that the well-being of a person does not rely on physical health alone. It incorporates mental, physical, and spiritual health as a whole and divides people into three types or *doshas* (see pages 18–23). These *doshas* categorize people according to their energy patterns, mental attitudes, physical descriptions, and personal strengths and weaknesses. Each *dosha* type has a particular weakness toward certain disorders.

When environmental factors remain congenial to the individual, good physical, mental, and spiritual health will be maintained. But when factors change, if some unusual, inadequate, or excessive interaction between objects, senses, mind and body occurs, the three humors or energies gradually weaken and disease begins to afflict the body. These factors can be as diverse as climate change, misuse of the body, or psychological disturbances.

Prevention is better than cure

Yoga acts as a preventive measure to disease by reducing stress levels, keeping the internal organs toned and healthy and maintaining a balanced equilibrium between the physical, mental, and spiritual self. The emphasis is on unifying the system with a combination of breathing techniques, gentle exercise, and mind control. This produces a tranquillity that penetrates deep into the mind and soul. It affects the health of the person on all levels.

The gentle movement and deep stretching of yoga improves the circulation and releases the tension in the muscle group. Twisting and turning the body in all directions remove toxin build-up. Deep yoga breathing relaxes the nervous system and calms and soothes the brain while increasing oxygen levels. This purifies the blood and increases the blood supply to the internal organs, which replenishes and rejuvenates the cells.

Yoga also combats the aging process and the degenerative diseases that usually accompany old age. Arthritis, osteoporosis, and urinary and digestive disorders can be prevented by practicing yoga. Yoga is a valuable tool in boosting the entire immune system to help prevent ill health from occurring in all age groups.

RESPIRATION

Breath, or *prana*, is the life force. *Pranayama* is the science of breath control. In yoga, we learn the importance of inhalation, exhalation, and retention of the breath. Correct breathing rejuvenates the entire system by sending increased oxygen into the bloodstream to nourish and revitalize the internal organs. Yoga breathing acts as a natural tranquillizer for the nervous system. The deeper you breathe, the calmer the mind becomes. It is an automatic physical reaction to calm and soothe the brain.

Breathing with arms

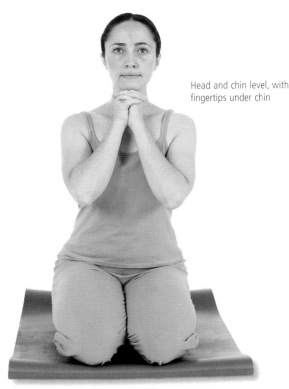

Head and chin level, with fingertips under chin

1 Sit on your heels with hands clasped under your chin. Make sure you keep your chin parallel to the ground.

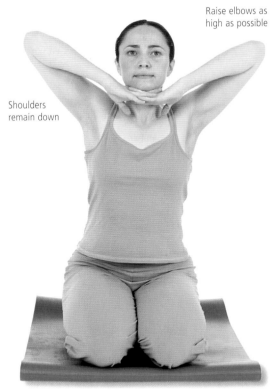

Raise elbows as high as possible

Shoulders remain down

2 Inhale for 6 seconds, and simultaneously lift your elbows up as high as possible. Do not bend forward. Keep your spine straight.

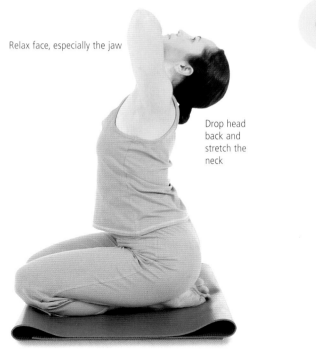

Relax face, especially the jaw

Drop head back and stretch the neck

3 Keeping the movements fluid, slowly exhale through your mouth as you look upward and drop your head backward.

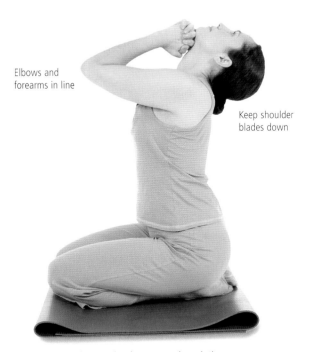

Elbows and forearms in line

Keep shoulder blades down

4 Continue to exhale through the mouth while you move your elbows together. Keep the fingers interlaced and knuckles against your chin. Drop your arms to your sides and rest for a moment. Repeat the exercise 10 times.

BENEFITS

Most people only breathe one-third of their full capacity. This exercise strengthens the lungs and teaches you how to fill the lungs to their full capacity. This improves circulation and energizes and rejuvenates the entire system. Always breathe through your nose from the diaphragm as you inhale and slowly exhale from the mouth. This method forces the mind to remain still and calm while curing respiratory disorders such as asthma, bronchitis, and emphysema.

Physical
• Promotes glowing complexion
• Improves posture

Mental
• Calms and soothes the nervous system
• Quiets the brain
• Provides clarity of thought

Health
• Cures breathing disorders
• Prevents panic attacks
• Prevents asthma
• Prevents bronchitis
• Prevents emphysema
• Improves circulation
• Cures lethargy

Ayurvedic
• Good for all *doshas*

Energy booster

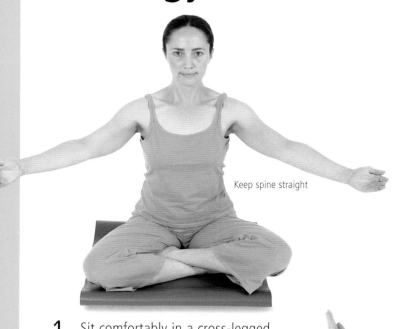

Keep spine straight

1 Sit comfortably in a cross-legged position on the floor, or upright in a chair with both feet flat on the floor. It is important that your spine stays straight and your head is in line with your neck and back. Concentrate on your navel and inhale deeply, taking your arms up slowly around your body. Feel the breath moving to fill your lungs.

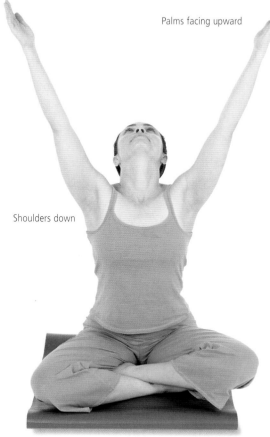

Palms facing upward

Shoulders down

2 Continuing to inhale, lift your arms up as you look upward.

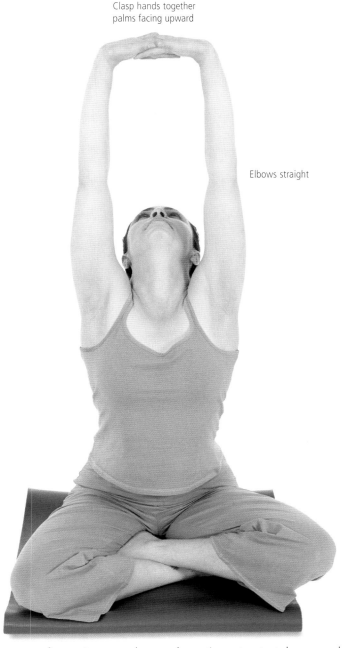

Clasp hands together
palms facing upward

Elbows straight

BENEFITS

Breath control is a valuable technique, not only to reduce stress levels but also to increase oxygen into the bloodstream. This rejuvenates and replenishes every cell and nerve in the body. It is important to fill the lungs to their full capacity to boost energy levels and help prevent breathing problems. Breathing deeply acts as a natural tranquilizer for the nervous system. The deeper you breathe, the calmer the mind becomes.

Physical
• Improves posture
• Has anti-aging effects
• Releases tension in neck and shoulders

Mental
• Calms and soothes the brain
• Provides clarity of thought

Health
• Prevents panic attacks
• Prevents breathing disorders
• Cures lethargy
• Improves circulation
• Rejuvenates cells

Ayurvedic
• Good for *Kapha* types

3   Clasp your fingertips together and continue to stretch upward. Exhale, and drop your head back, releasing your hands in a burst of energy. Repeat this exercise 5 to 10 times.

DIGESTION

Many yoga postures aid digestion because of the unique mixture of turning and twisting of the body in different directions. We cannot massage the internal organs, but by putting pressure on certain areas, combined with deep breathing, we can tone and replenish the liver, kidneys, and spleen. Toxins build up in the system and it is important to release these poisonous substances that can weaken and eventually harm the whole body.

Modified bow

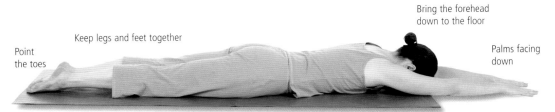

Point the toes

Keep legs and feet together

Bring the forehead down to the floor

Palms facing down

1 Lie on your stomach on the floor with your legs together and arms outstretched in front of you, your palms facing down. Point your toes.

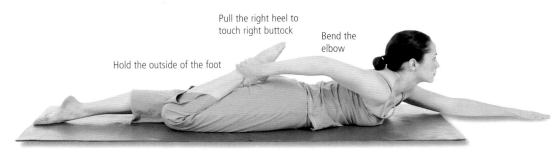

Pull the right heel to touch right buttock

Bend the elbow

Hold the outside of the foot

2 Inhale, and bend your right leg. Hold on to your foot with your right hand and pull your heel down toward your right buttock. Exhale, and hold briefly to feel the stretch in the hamstring.

BENEFITS

This pose increases the pressure on the abdominal wall, which massages and invigorates the internal organs—especially the digestive tract. It is essentially a backbend, so all the muscles in the back are strengthened and toned. It improves the elasticity and flexibility of the spine, and promotes youthfulness. It is a total stretch for the spine, so when you practice this pose regularly, you will feel energized and dynamic. Although this is a wonderful exercise to prepare for pregnancy, do not do this pose while pregnant because it puts too much pressure on the uterus.

Physical
- Flattens stomach
- Tightens buttocks muscles
- Stretches neck
- Increases circulation to face
- Increases suppleness and youthfulness
- Increases energy levels

Mental
- Improves mental balance and harmony
- Improves concentration
- Increases determination

Health
- Massages internal organs
- Aids digestion
- Helps asthma and other respiratory problems
- Relieves menstrual problems
- Helps bladder, kidney, and spleen to function properly
- Alleviates back pain
- Helps irritable bowel syndrome and other bowel disorders
- Alleviates fatigue and lethargy

Ayurvedic
- Good for *Vata* types

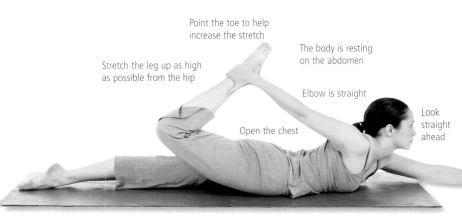

Point the toe to help increase the stretch

The body is resting on the abdomen

Stretch the leg up as high as possible from the hip

Elbow is straight

Open the chest

Look straight ahead

3 Inhale and stretch your leg up to create a bow shape. Keep your left leg and hip on the floor. Look upward, but do not strain your neck.

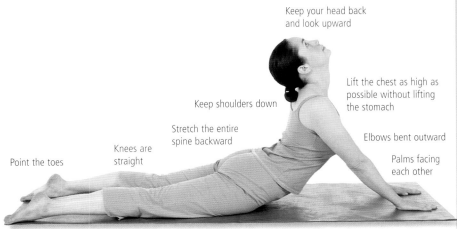

Keep your head back and look upward

Keep shoulders down

Lift the chest as high as possible without lifting the stomach

Stretch the entire spine backward

Knees are straight

Point the toes

Elbows bent outward

Palms facing each other

4 Release your leg and return to the start position, then take both arms out in front of you with palms facing and with your elbows turned outward. Inhale, pushing both palms into the floor, and raise your chest, looking upward. Keep your hipbones down, and tighten the buttock muscles. Exhale, and come back to the start position. Repeat the exercise on the other side.

DIGESTION: MODIFIED BOW

BACK PAIN

As stress manifests in the body, many people are prone to back pain and chronic conditions such as lumbago and sciatica. It is necessary first to relieve the pain and then build the muscles in the lower back to stop the pain from recurring. Yoga exercise provides a natural solution because of the emphasis on posture and alignment. Mental relaxation also helps eliminate nervous tension that becomes trapped in the muscles of the back.

Cat

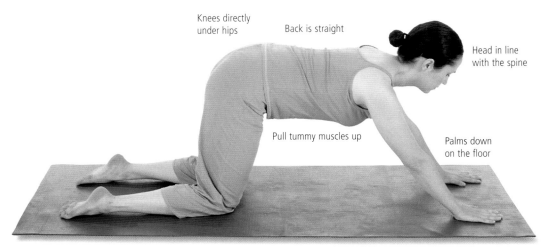

Knees directly under hips

Back is straight

Head in line with the spine

Pull tummy muscles up

Palms down on the floor

1 Kneel on all fours with straight arms, keeping your knees under your hips and your hands in front of your head.

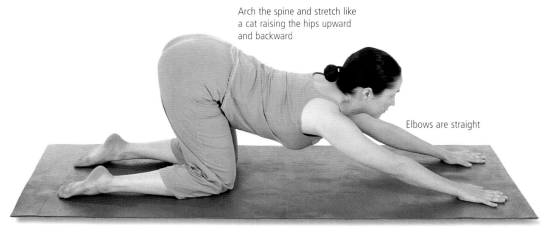

Arch the spine and stretch like a cat raising the hips upward and backward

Elbows are straight

2 Inhale deeply, and push down on your palms, so that you can lift your hips upward into a kneeling position, just like a cat.

BENEFITS

When stress and anxiety lock the back muscles, it is necessary to release the tension accumulated in the spine. This is a gentle and effective way to relieve back pain by combining deep breathing with the movement. The position of the forehead on the floor also calms and soothes the brain, so people who also suffer from headaches will also benefit. This exercise is a quick fix because as soon as you curve the spine forward you will feel the pain disappear. It also slows down the pulse rate and regulates your breathing pattern.

Physical
• Improves posture

Mental
• Calms the mind
• Soothes the brain
• Enhances inner peace
• Has a feel-good factor

Health
• Releases back pain
• Releases stress in the central nervous system
• Relieves headaches
• Lowers pulse rate
• Boosts mental health

Ayurvedic
• Particularly good for *Pitta* and *Kapha* types

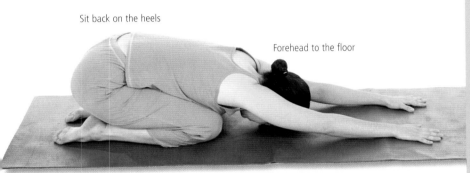

Sit back on the heels

Forehead to the floor

3 Exhale, and stretch your hips back so that you sit on your heels. Straighten your elbows, stretching your arms out in front of you. Place your forehead on the floor. Breathe normally and relax.

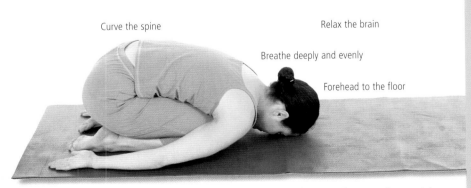

Curve the spine

Relax the brain

Breathe deeply and evenly

Forehead to the floor

4 Take your arms back, so your hands are in line with your feet with palms facing up, and breathe deeply to relax the brain.

Back twist

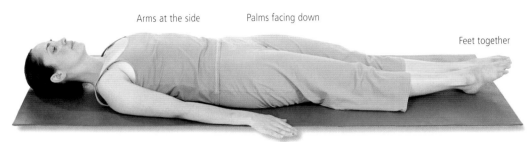

Arms at the side   Palms facing down

Feet together

1 Lie flat on the floor and place your arms on either side. Palms should face down. Relax the body, inhale and exhale deeply for 10 counts.

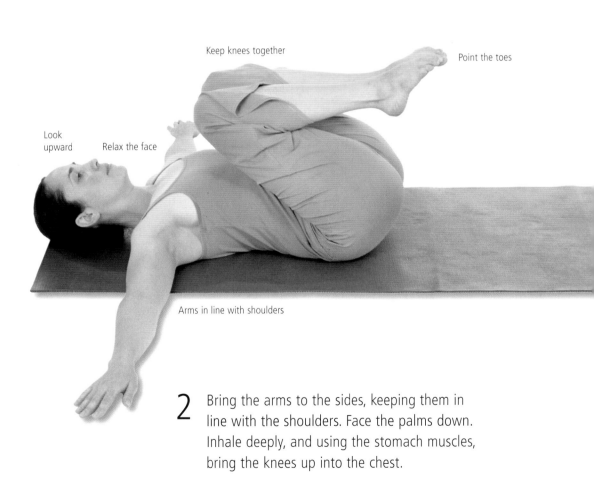

Keep knees together

Point the toes

Look upward   Relax the face

Arms in line with shoulders

2 Bring the arms to the sides, keeping them in line with the shoulders. Face the palms down. Inhale deeply, and using the stomach muscles, bring the knees up into the chest.

BENEFITS

People who suffer from back pain believe wrongly that they should not move or exercise during an attack. Yoga provides a perfect solution because it teaches that the first step is to alleviate the pain and the second step is to build the muscles in the lower back to prevent further pain from recurring. This gentle twist does both. It relaxes the entire spinal column, which releases the pain immediately, and it also strengthens the abdominal muscles to prevent more serious back ailments like sciatica and lumbago from manifesting. When the knees pull up into the chest, the tension in the lower back ceases, and during the twist, the neck, shoulders, and upper and lower back are fully stretched.

Physical
- Flattens stomach
- Strengthens the abdominal muscles
- Improves flexibility
- Increases suppleness of the spine

Mental
- Promotes inner calm

Health
- Alleviates back pain
- Prevents sciatica and lumbago
- Destresses nervous system

Look over the opposite shoulder

Keep the shoulder down on the floor

Bring the knees as close to the arm as possible to increase the stretch

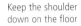
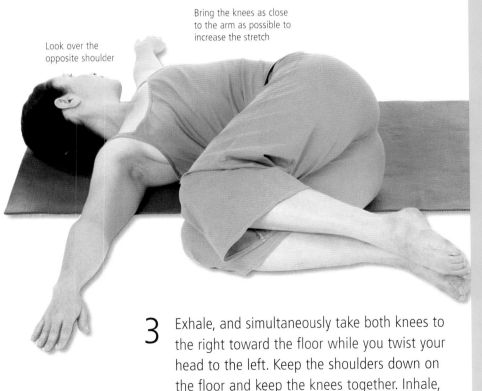

3 Exhale, and simultaneously take both knees to the right toward the floor while you twist your head to the left. Keep the shoulders down on the floor and keep the knees together. Inhale, bring the knees up into the chest as close as possible, exhale, and twist to the other side. Repeat 5 times to each side.

NECK & SHOULDER PAIN

Most people feel tension and stress in the neck, shoulders, and upper back. Yoga is an effective way to release pain, combining movement with mental relaxation. There is a difference between good pain and bad pain. If you feel dull pain, continue with a movement, but if it becomes sharp, stop at once so you don't aggravate the condition. Yoga is gentle with concentrated emphasis on what you are doing and experiencing.

Shoulder shrugs

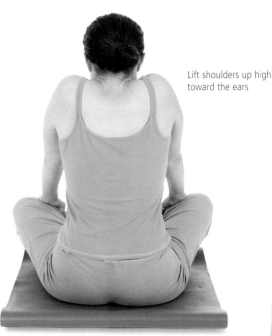

Lift shoulders up high toward the ears

1 Sitting cross-legged on the floor, inhale and take your shoulders up high toward your ears.

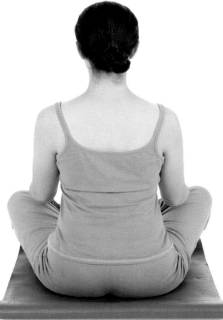

Keep head in line with back

2 As you exhale, drop your shoulders down and push your shoulder blades together, opening out your chest. Repeat a few times until the stiffness starts to leave your body. Breathe deeply to help shift the tightness.

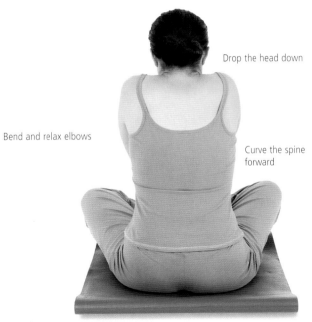

Drop the head down

Bend and relax elbows

Curve the spine forward

3 Inhale, and take the shoulders forward and drop the head down to create more space for the shoulders.

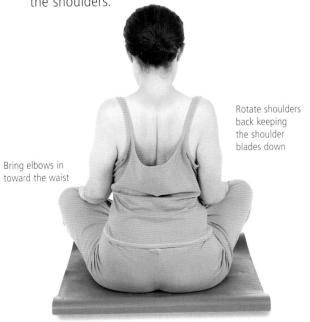

Rotate shoulders back keeping the shoulder blades down

Bring elbows in toward the waist

4 As you exhale, move your shoulders back in a circular motion. To repeat the exercise, inhale, and take your shoulders forward and up, then exhale, taking them back and down. Keep all your movements fluid and graceful. Return to the start position. As you exercise, keep still, concentrating on your neck and shoulders.

BENEFITS

When people are very stressed, tension accumulates into specific muscle groups, especially the neck and shoulders. This exercise gently releases the stiffness by combining movement with yoga breathing. As you exaggerate the movement upward, inhale and concentrate on the tension, and as you exhale, imagine that all the muscular tension is leaving the body. Visualizing tension and then releasing it with the breath is a valuable technique that can be used to release stress in all parts of the body.

Physical
• Improves posture

Mental
• Focuses attention
• Improves concentration
• Releases mental stress

Health
• Releases stress in muscles
• Calms the nervous system
• Soothes the nerves
• Relaxes the brain

Head rolls

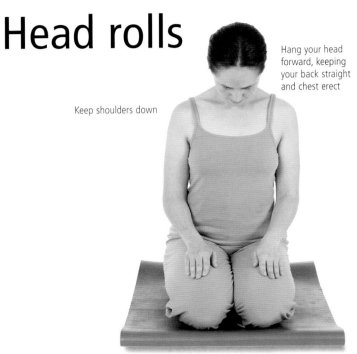

Hang your head forward, keeping your back straight and chest erect

Keep shoulders down

1 Kneeling or sitting tall in perfect posture, begin the head rolls with your head in correct alignment to your neck and back. Drop your chin down onto your chest.

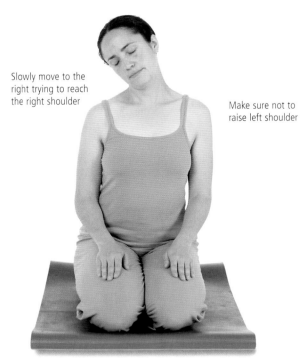

Slowly move to the right trying to reach the right shoulder

Make sure not to raise left shoulder

2 Inhale deeply and slowly roll your head in a circular pattern to your right shoulder.

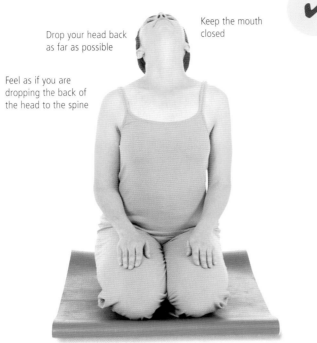

Drop your head back as far as possible

Keep the mouth closed

Feel as if you are dropping the back of the head to the spine

3 Continuing to inhale, drop your head all the way back as far as possible without moving your shoulders and upper body.

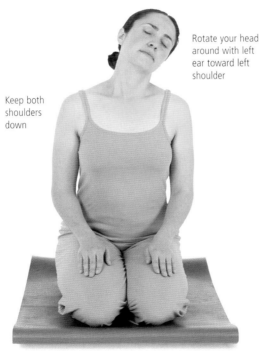

Rotate your head around with left ear toward left shoulder

Keep both shoulders down

4 Slowly exhale, and bend your head toward your left shoulder, then slowly bring your chin back down to your chest. Repeat the head roll clockwise and then two more times counterclockwise.

BENEFITS

This exercise is an excellent way to release tension not only in the neck and shoulders but also in the upper and middle back. Using the breath, as you inhale and exhale, feel where the stiffness is. When you locate the exact position, as you move your head in a circle, stop and visualize the tension leaving the body. There is a tendency not to complete a full circle but to perform it halfway due to pain. If you feel a sharp pain, stop at once. Otherwise, keep the body stationary so the head can move freely around.

Physical
- Improves posture
- Relaxes face

Mental
- Improves mental concentration
- Aids visualization
- Focuses the mind

Health
- Releases blocked energy
- Relaxes the brain
- Calms and soothes the nervous system

WOMEN'S PROBLEMS

Many women suffer from hormone imbalances, which cause mood swings, irritable behavior, and emotional stress. Fertility can become an issue, and the more you try to become pregnant the more difficult it can become. Yoga tones the ovaries and uterus, and the inverted poses stabilize the thyroid and control the metabolism. This reduces cravings and helps maintain a steady weight. Correct breathing calms the nerves, so you are relaxed and able to cope with the stresses and strains of modern living.

Cobra

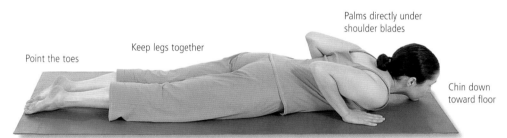

Point the toes

Keep legs together

Palms directly under shoulder blades

Chin down toward floor

1 Lie flat on your stomach with your feet together. Point your toes, bend your arms close to your body, and place your palms flat under your shoulder blades. Point your chin downward.

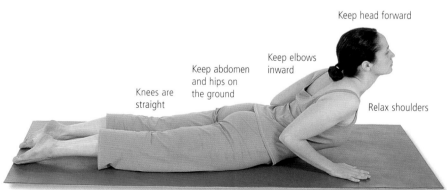

Keep head forward

Keep elbows inward

Keep abdomen and hips on the ground

Knees are straight

Relax shoulders

2 Inhale, and raise your head off the floor. Place your hands on the floor with your elbows pointing inward. Keep your chin up, and make sure your hip bones stay on the floor. Breathe normally and hold for 10 seconds. On the last exhalation, slowly lower yourself to the floor and return to Step 1. Repeat.

BENEFITS

This position is called the Cobra because the body resembles a snake poised to strike. The entire spine is being stretched upward with the gravity on the pubis and sacrum. This movement stimulates and tones the uterus and ovaries, which helps women with fertility problems. It also strengthens the lower back, which helps with carrying extra weight during pregnancy. It is also an excellent post-natal exercise to send fresh oxygen and blood supply to the ovaries after childbirth. It also helps regulate the menstrual cycle and helps the thyroid work more effectively.

Physical
- Tones legs and buttocks
- Stretches neck muscles
- Has anti-aging effects
- Improves posture
- Increases flexibility and suppleness of the spine

Mental
- Improves concentration
- Focuses the mind

Health
- Prevents back pain
- Alleviates back problems
- Tones uterus and ovaries
- Regulates menstrual cycle
- Increases effectiveness of thyroid and adrenal glands

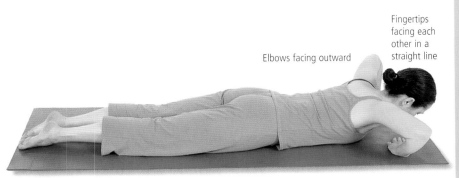

Elbows facing outward

Fingertips facing each other in a straight line

3 Return to Step 1, but this time place your hands under the breastbone and point your elbows outward.

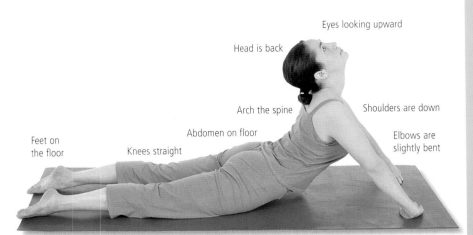

Eyes looking upward

Head is back

Arch the spine

Shoulders are down

Abdomen on floor

Feet on the floor

Knees straight

Elbows are slightly bent

4 Inhale, push down and lift your body off the floor. Look upward, keeping your shoulders down and your hips just off the floor. Breathing normally, hold for 10 seconds. On the last exhalation, slowly lower yourself and relax.

Shoulder stand

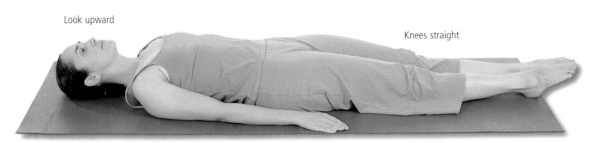

Look upward

Knees straight

1 Lie on the floor, legs outstretched and arms at your side. Palms facing down. Point your toes.

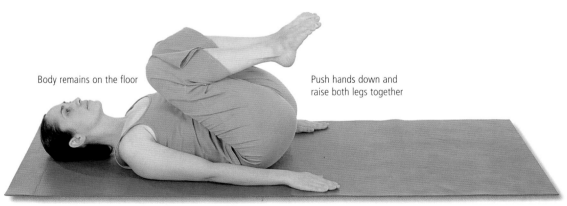

Body remains on the floor

Push hands down and raise both legs together

2 Inhale deeply, pushing your palms down, while bringing your knees up to your chest. Keep pushing your palms down and lift your spine off the floor.

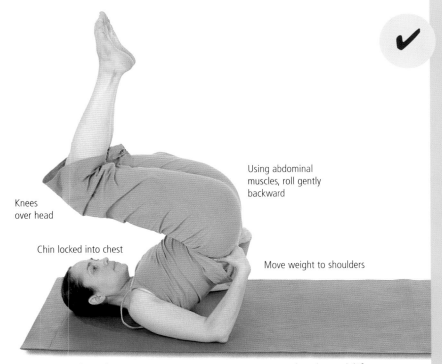

Knees over head

Chin locked into chest

Using abdominal muscles, roll gently backward

Move weight to shoulders

3 Place your hands on your waist to support your back and lift your legs up.

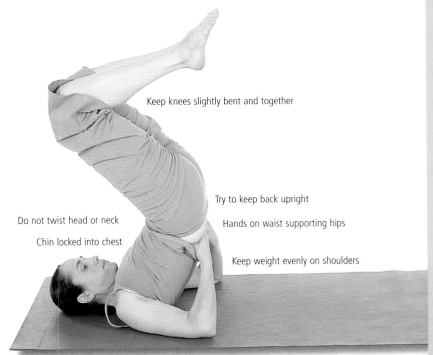

Keep knees slightly bent and together

Do not twist head or neck

Chin locked into chest

Try to keep back upright

Hands on waist supporting hips

Keep weight evenly on shoulders

4 Lock your chin into your chest. Exhale, and breathe normally while holding this position. Try to hold still for 30 to 60 seconds. To come down, inhale, and while exhaling, slowly lower your back and legs to the floor. Keep breathing deeply and evenly.

BENEFITS

This exercise in yoga is called the Queen's pose because of the direct benefit to women and their health problems. It is an inverted posture that sends fresh oxygen and blood supply to all the female organs. In this position, as the blood flows downward, all the cells are being replenished and oxygenated. The chin presses into the throat, which stimulates the thyroid gland and balances hormones. This regulates the menstrual cycle and weight fluctuations. It also regulates mood swings and helps prevent depression.

Physical
- Increases flexibility
- Increases suppleness of spine

Mental
- Prevents mood swings
- Calms the mind

Health
- Balances hormones
- Regulates thyroid gland
- Relieves varicose veins
- Tones uterus and ovaries
- Prevents depression
- Helps insomnia
- Relieves menstrual pain and regulates the menstrual cycle

Ayurvedic
- Good for all *doshas*

METABOLISM
Plough

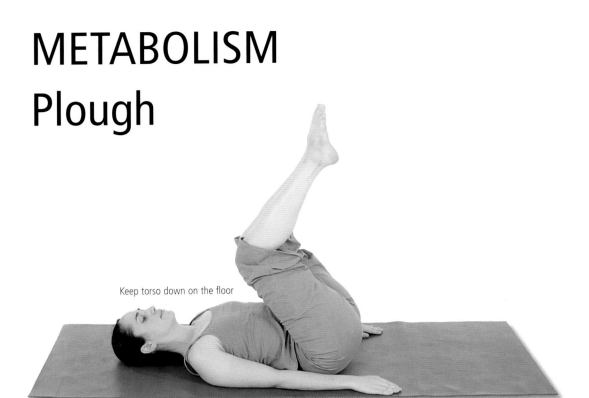

Keep torso down on the floor

1 Lie flat on the floor with your arms on either side. Inhale, and bring the knees into the chest.

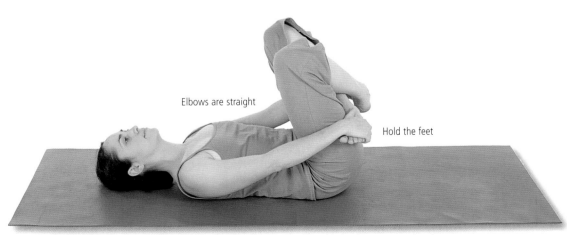

Elbows are straight

Hold the feet

2 Cross the ankles and hold on to the toes while bringing the knees closer into the chest.

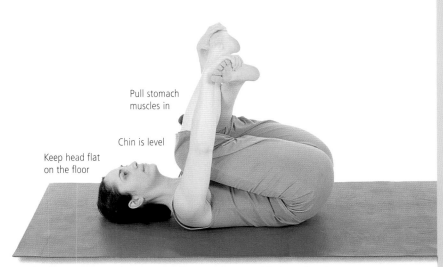

Pull stomach
muscles in

Chin is level

Keep head flat
on the floor

3 Inhale, contract the stomach muscles and bring the knees as close as possible into the chest.

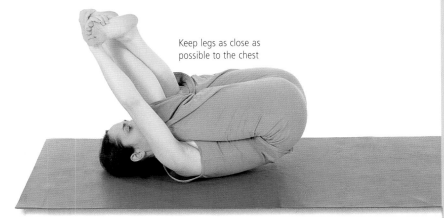

Keep legs as close as possible to the chest

4 Bring the legs slowly over your head and roll back onto the top of the spine.

continued ▶

BENEFITS

As we age, the metabolism naturally slows down. The result is weight gain and what is commonly known as middle-age spread. This exercise helps regulate the metabolism and hormone imbalances because of the position of the head, neck, throat, and chest. It is an inverted posture that takes the legs over the head. This relieves menstrual cramps and sends fresh blood supply to all the internal organs. This nourishes and replenishes the cells and improves blood circulation in general.

Physical
- Promotes youthful appearance
- Increases flexibility
- Increases suppleness of spine
- Improves posture
- Releases muscular tension
- Tones abdominal muscles and legs

Mental
- Promotes inner calm
- Promotes mental relaxation
- Soothes the brain
- Calms the nervous system
- Promotes inner balance and mental poise

Health
- Improves circulation
- Aids indigestion
- Cures constipation
- Regulates thyroid
- Replenishes internal organs
- Relieves insomnia
- Balances hormones

METABOLISM: PLOUGH

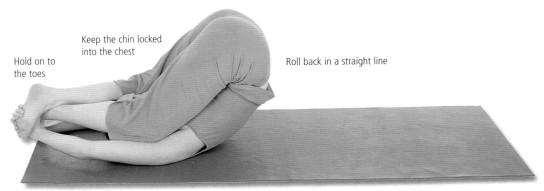

Hold on to
the toes

Keep the chin locked
into the chest

Roll back in a straight line

5 Continue to roll backward and balance on the shoulders. Exhale,
breathe normally, and hold for 5 counts.

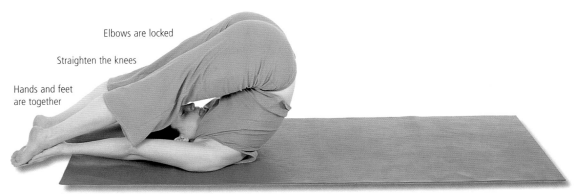

Elbows are locked

Straighten the knees

Hands and feet
are together

6 Roll back on to the shoulders and straighten the legs behind you.
Uncross the ankles, and keep stretching the legs so the chin is
locked in to the chest. Breathe normally and hold for 5 counts.

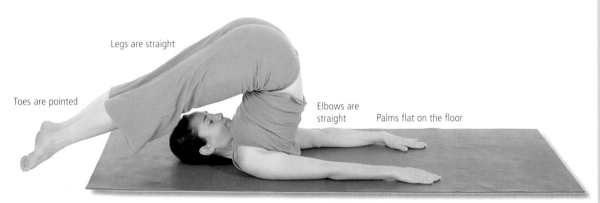

Legs are straight

Toes are pointed

Elbows are straight

Palms flat on the floor

7 Lift the feet slightly off the floor, release the arms forward, and hold
   the pose. Hold for 5 counts.

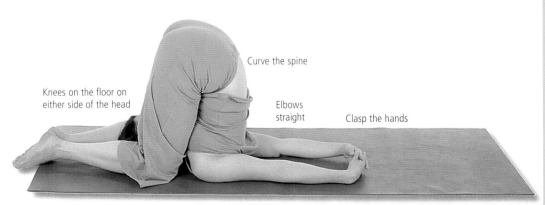

Curve the spine

Knees on the floor on
either side of the head

Elbows
straight

Clasp the hands

8 Relax the spine and drop the knees down to the floor. Clasp the
   hands in front of you. Breathe normally, hold for at least 10–15
   counts.

CIRCULATION & HEART

Many people lead sedentary lives and complain of fatigue and low energy. This affects self-esteem and can lead to depression. Especially as we age, it is vital to exercise the heart and boost circulation. Yoga exercise is the best way to increase energy and improve health by combining deep breathing with stretching and twisting in all directions. This action rejuvenates each cell, nerve, and muscle in the body and prolongs good health.

Side stretch 2

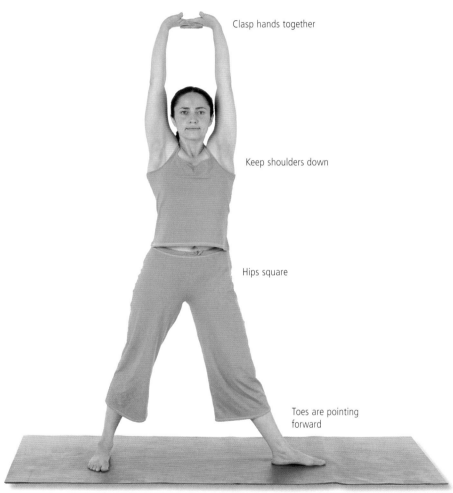

Clasp hands together

Keep shoulders down

Hips square

Toes are pointing forward

1 Stand up straight with your feet 3–4 ft (1–1.2 m) apart, toes pointing forward. Clasp your hands together and stretch your arms above your head as high as possible. Keep your shoulders down and elbows straight. Inhale and exhale deeply and evenly as you exercise.

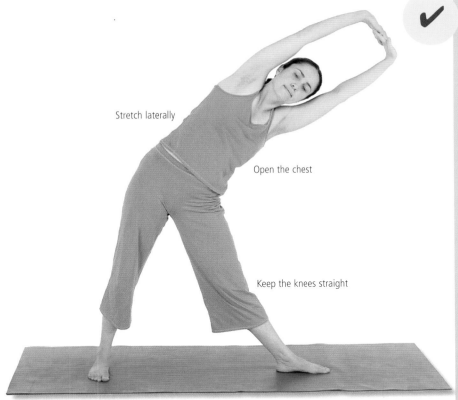

Stretch laterally

Open the chest

Keep the knees straight

2 Begin to stretch sideways to the left from the waist.

BENEFITS

By taking deep and even breaths while stretching, you send fresh oxygen into the system, and this boosts your circulation. As the movement becomes more difficult, the breath will quicken and the pulse rate increase. This is precisely the time to deepen the breath so it stays even. Stretching the arms over the head will stimulate the heart rate and increase energy levels. Stretching sideways keeps the body supple and flexible and increases the mobility of the spine.

Physical
• Trims waist
• Boosts energy levels
• Increases flexibility of the spine

Mental
• Calms the brain

Health
• Improves circulation
• Promotes lymph drainage
• Lubricates the joints
• Alleviates back pain

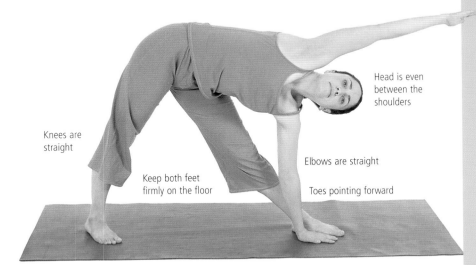

Head is even between the shoulders

Knees are straight

Keep both feet firmly on the floor

Elbows are straight

Toes pointing forward

3 Release your left arm, lower it to your knee, and hold this position for a few seconds. Move your left hand down, place it on the floor with the palm flat, keeping your arm and hips in a straight line. Hold this for 10 seconds. Release the stretch, stand up straight and repeat the exercise on the other side. If you cannot touch the floor, grip your left ankle with your left hand.

Deep lunge balance

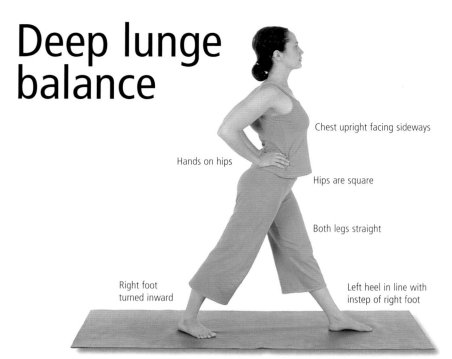

Chest upright facing sideways

Hands on hips

Hips are square

Both legs straight

Right foot turned inward

Left heel in line with instep of right foot

1 Stand upright with your feet 3–4 ft (1–1.2 m) apart, facing forward. Turn your right foot to the right so that the instep is in line with the left heel. Turn your upper body so that your hips are square and your breastbone is in line with your knee.

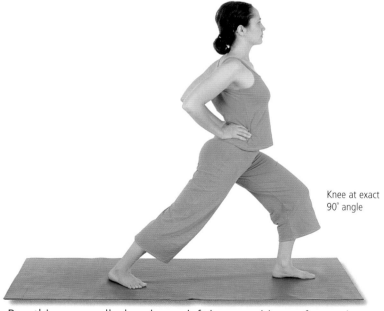

Knee at exact 90° angle

2 Breathing normally, bend your left knee and lunge forward.

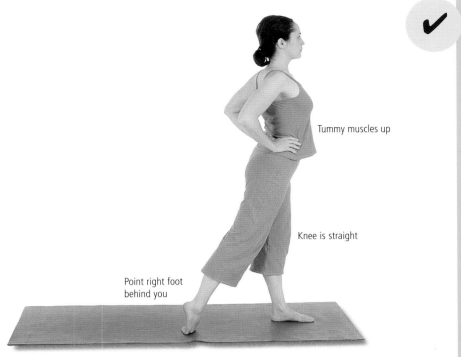

Tummy muscles up

Knee is straight

Point right foot behind you

3 Straighten both legs, point your right foot behind you, and focus on one spot on the floor to prepare to balance.

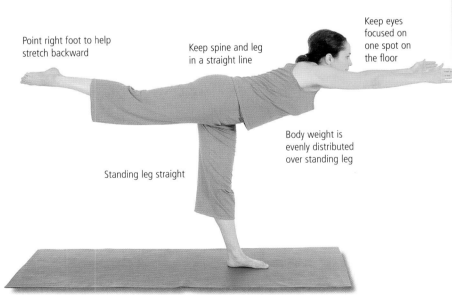

Point right foot to help stretch backward

Keep spine and leg in a straight line

Keep eyes focused on one spot on the floor

Body weight is evenly distributed over standing leg

Standing leg straight

4 Inhale deeply, and lift your right leg off the floor as you bend forward. Exhale, and breathe normally as you straighten both legs, while keeping your shoulders and hips in a straight line. Hold for as long as possible and bend your left knee to finish. Return to the start position and repeat the exercise on the other side.

BENEFITS

This exercise increases circulation while improving concentration and balance. Balancing exercises take up more energy than you can imagine because of the deep concentration. As you balance on one leg, the pulse increases, which stimulates and exercises the heart muscle. This is a challenging pose. Before you begin the exercise, visualize yourself in the final position exactly balancing without shaking or moving from one side to another.

Physical
- Tones buttocks, legs, and abdominal muscles
- Builds stamina
- Builds muscular strength

Mental
- Focuses the mind
- Improves concentration
- Increases willpower

Health
- Improves circulation

Ayurvedic
- Good for *Kapha* types

yoga for stress-relief & relaxation

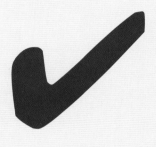

Yoga is a holistic concept that teaches us how to integrate the mind, body, and spiritual self. Only when these energies are united can mental balance and inner peace be found. In these confusing and chaotic times, we all need to learn to cope with uncertainties and fears. Yoga provides the perfect solution because it teaches us how to draw the energies inward in order to find positive solutions to difficult problems.

Whether it has to deal with family, jobs, or relationships, yoga helps you to find inner balance with the ability to relax on all levels. When people are nervous and irritable, they become unreasonable and are unable to seek truth and wisdom. It is often said that some people cannot see the woods for the trees or on a deeper level are unable to see or understand the real meaning of their own existence. Remaining calm and relaxed with clarity of mind and thoughts should be the goal of all students of yoga.

Purification

Panchakarma is the ancient *Ayurvedic* method of purification and rejuvenation. It consists of delicately balanced physical cleansings that also lend greater clarity to our mind, help to balance our emotions, and enhance our spiritual practice. Done properly and for a sufficient length of time, it is a powerful force for the prevention of health problems and for rejuvenation of the body. This method has been growing in popularity, and clinical studies have found that *Panchakarma* balances biochemistry, improves cardiovascular risk factors, and, by reducing free radicals, strengthens immunity, increases joint flexibility, and slows the aging process.

It also has a profound balancing and soothing effect on one's emotional state. People who suffer from stress-related ailments and illnesses need to find a solution to restore harmony and balance. Every individual is assessed differently and a combination of diet, effective herbal remedies, and detoxifying therapies is prescribed. Spiritual counseling is also provided in order to restore balance and happiness to your mind and body.

Maintaining perfect health

According to *Ayurvedic* medicine, there are 5 elements to perfect health:
1) The digestive fire (*agni*) is in a balanced condition.
2) The body humors (*doshas*), *Vata*, *Pitta,* and *Kapha*, are in equilibrium.
3) The 3 waste products (urine, feces, and sweat) are produced and
   eliminated normally.
4) The 7 bodily tissues and all the organs are functioning normally.
5) The mind, senses, and the consciousness are working harmoniously
   together.

When the balance of these systems is disturbed, disease begins. The wrong lifestyle or diet, negative or repressed emotions, or stress factors can throw the delicate balance of the *doshas* off center. When any of the three is aggravated, the gastric fire (digestive capacity) is affected. As a result, toxins are produced that enter the bloodstream and circulate throughout the body. This clogs the energy meridians, or *chakras*, causing retention of the toxins in the body. Once the body's toxic level reaches a certain height, the vital life energy (*prana*) is diminished, weakening the immune system and affecting the cell metabolic energy immediately. Yoga practice unifies all these systems by making sure that the physical, mental, emotional, and spiritual Selves are working in unison.

Balancing workout

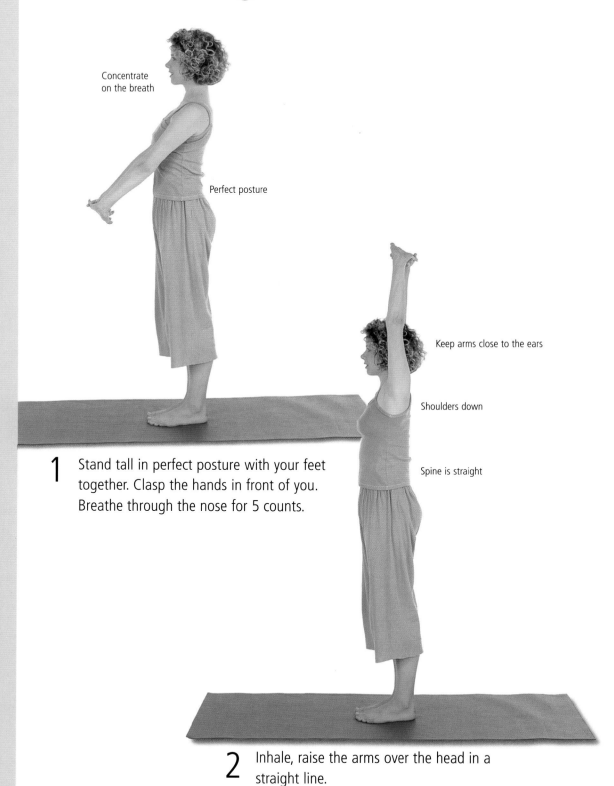

Concentrate on the breath

Perfect posture

Keep arms close to the ears

Shoulders down

Spine is straight

1 Stand tall in perfect posture with your feet together. Clasp the hands in front of you. Breathe through the nose for 5 counts.

2 Inhale, raise the arms over the head in a straight line.

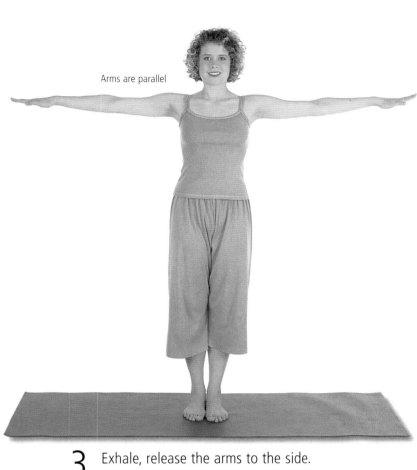

Arms are parallel

3 Exhale, release the arms to the side.

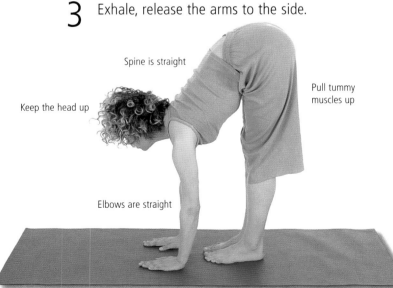

Spine is straight

Keep the head up

Pull tummy muscles up

Elbows are straight

4 Bring the arms in front of you, lean forward and place the palms of the hands on the floor.

continued ▶

BENEFITS

Yoga is a nonviolent system of movement that is based on a holistic approach to health. These physical movements increase circulation and stimulate the endocrine glands, which also balances the distribution of hormones, blood circulation, lymph return, and energy flow to the nervous system. Yoga movements exercise the muscles and joints, which keeps the connective tissue healthy and pliable. This balancing workout brings the mental, physical, emotional, and spiritual self together as a whole and focuses on restoring harmony and inner peace.

Physical
- Tones the whole body
- Promotes a glowing complexion
- Trims the waist
- Tightens the buttocks
- Improves flexibility

Mental
- Promotes inner calm
- Promotes inner poise
- Calms the brain

Health
- Increases circulation
- Increases oxygen to the blood supply
- Destresses nervous system

Ayurvedic
- Balances all *doshas*

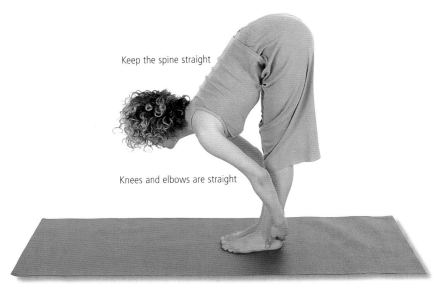

Keep the spine straight

Knees and elbows are straight

5 Keeping your spine in the same position, take hold of your ankles.

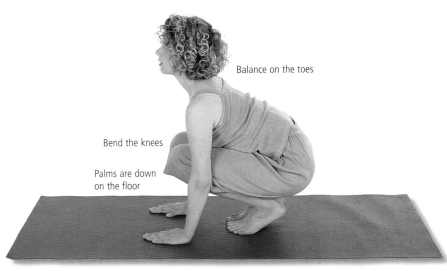

Balance on the toes

Bend the knees

Palms are down on the floor

6 Bend the knees, balance on the toes, and place the palms down on the floor.

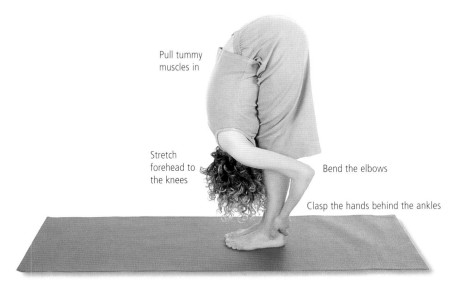

Pull tummy
muscles in

Stretch
forehead to
the knees

Bend the elbows

Clasp the hands behind the ankles

7 Straighten your legs, place your feet firmly on the ground, and draw your body toward your legs trying to rest your upper body on the legs. Breathe normally, and hold for 5 counts.

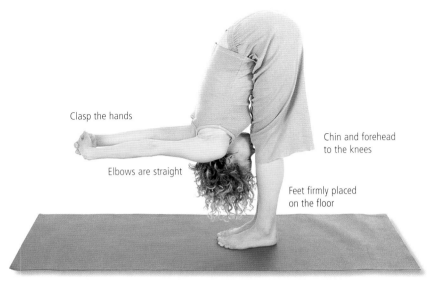

Clasp the hands

Elbows are straight

Chin and forehead
to the knees

Feet firmly placed
on the floor

8 Keeping your head down to your knees, clasp your hands in front of you, keeping your elbows straight. Breathe normally for 5 counts.

continued ▶

BALANCING WORKOUT

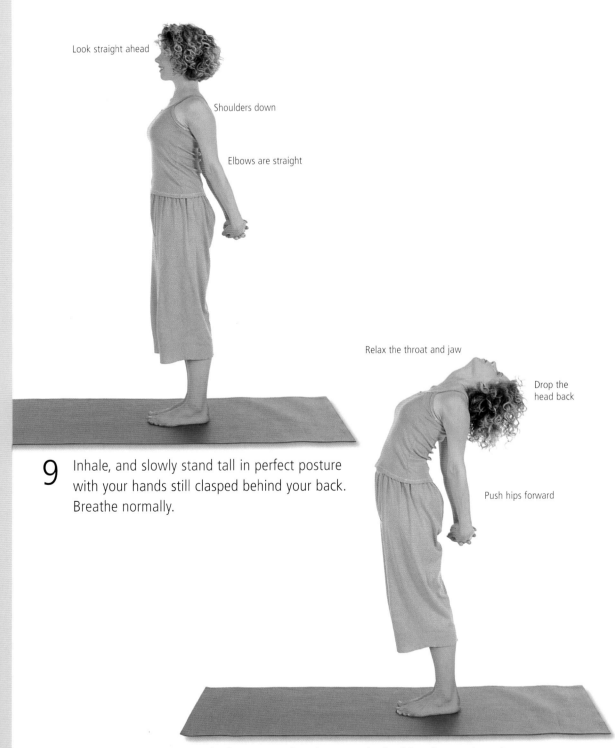

Look straight ahead

Shoulders down

Elbows are straight

Relax the throat and jaw

Drop the head back

Push hips forward

9 Inhale, and slowly stand tall in perfect posture with your hands still clasped behind your back. Breathe normally.

10 Open the chest, push the hips forward, and drop the head back as far as possible. Relax the throat and jaw.

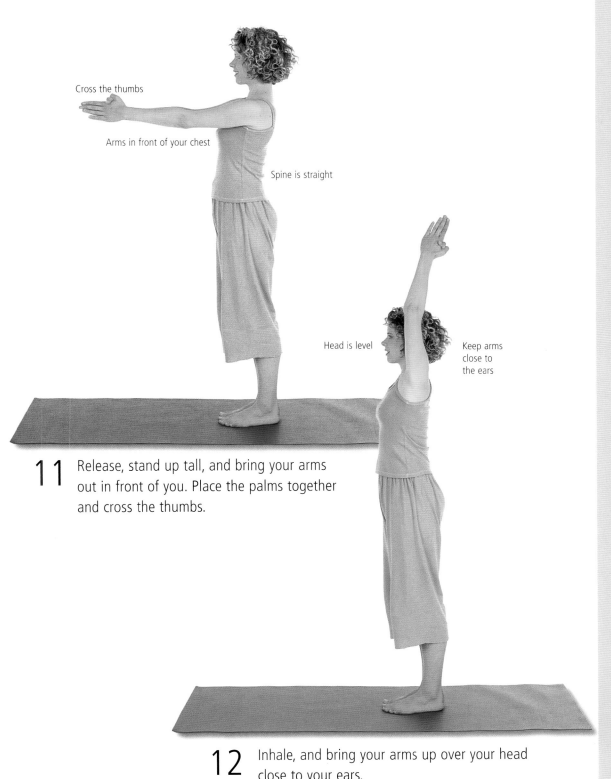

Cross the thumbs

Arms in front of your chest

Spine is straight

Head is level

Keep arms close to the ears

11 Release, stand up tall, and bring your arms out in front of you. Place the palms together and cross the thumbs.

12 Inhale, and bring your arms up over your head close to your ears.

continued ▶

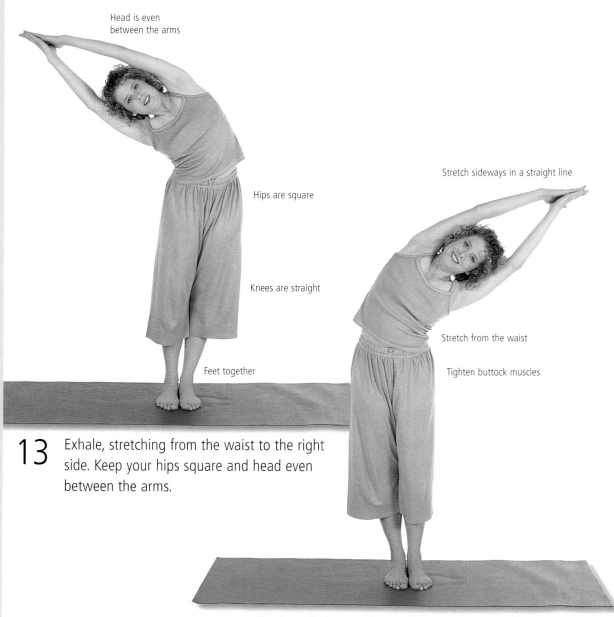

Head is even
between the arms

Hips are square

Knees are straight

Feet together

Stretch sideways in a straight line

Stretch from the waist

Tighten buttock muscles

13 Exhale, stretching from the waist to the right
side. Keep your hips square and head even
between the arms.

14 Inhale, standing tall as in Step 12, exhale, and
repeat Step 13 on the other side.

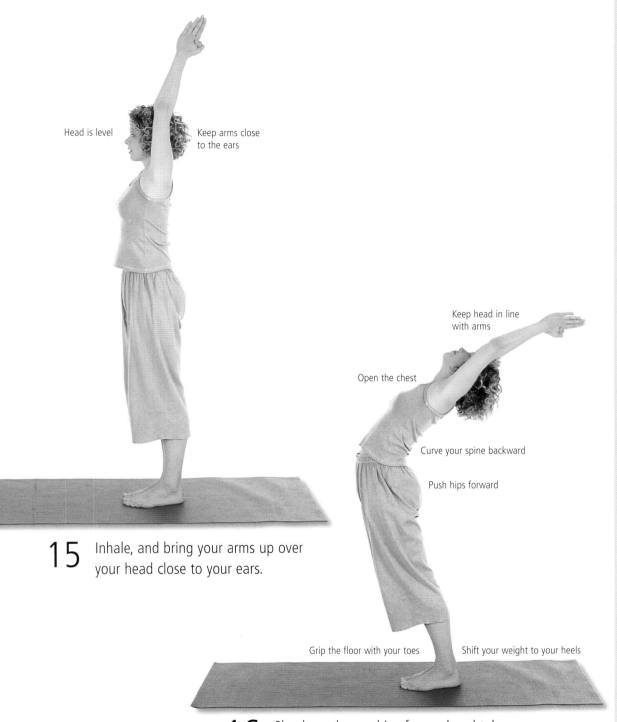

Head is level

Keep arms close to the ears

15 Inhale, and bring your arms up over your head close to your ears.

Keep head in line with arms

Open the chest

Curve your spine backward

Push hips forward

Grip the floor with your toes

Shift your weight to your heels

16 Slowly push your hips forward and take your weight onto your heels. Keep your knees straight and curve your spine backward into a back bend. Keep your head in line with your spine and your arms close to your ears. Inhale and exhale deeply and evenly, and try to hold for at least 5–10 counts.

Tree

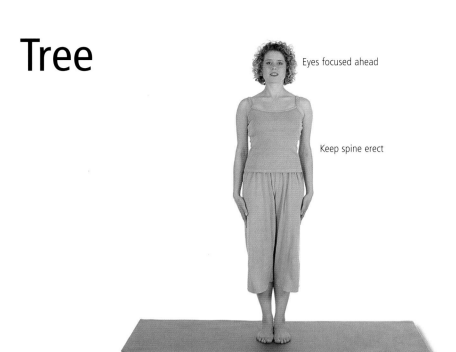

Eyes focused ahead

Keep spine erect

1 Stand tall in perfect posture with your arms to the side. Inhale and exhale, and begin to concentrate your mind. Focus straight ahead.

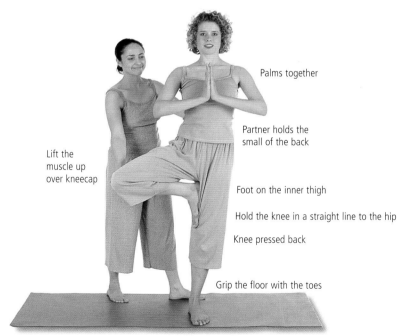

Palms together

Partner holds the small of the back

Lift the muscle up over kneecap

Foot on the inner thigh

Hold the knee in a straight line to the hip

Knee pressed back

Grip the floor with the toes

2 With your partner behind you to help you balance, bring the right foot up to the right inner thigh. Bring your palms together in front of your chest. Your partner should hold your right knee level so the hips remain square and have the other hand behind your back or on your shoulder to help you steady the pose. Breathe normally, and hold for 10 counts.

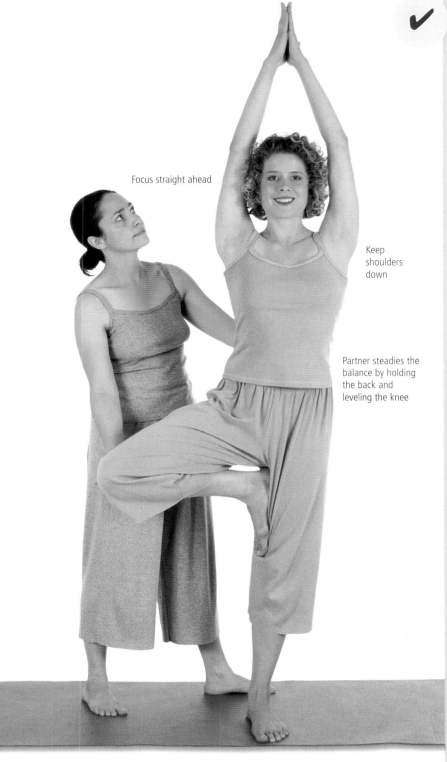

Focus straight ahead

Keep shoulders down

Partner steadies the balance by holding the back and leveling the knee

BENEFITS

All balancing exercises teach you how to focus the mind. This posture looks very simple, but in order to stand on one leg without moving takes intense concentration and physical effort. It is called the Tree because of the standing leg being rooted into the ground. When people are grounded or mentally and physically stable, they will remain rooted even through violent storms and chaos.

Physical
• Improves balance
• Improves posture

Mental
• Improves mental concentration
• Promotes single-mindedness
• Increases willpower

Health
• Promotes inner balance
• Promotes positive mental attitude

Ayurvedic
• Helps *Vata* types to focus and concentrate

3 With your partner holding you steady, inhale and stretch the arms over your head. Keep the palms together with your arms close to the ears. Exhale, breathe normally, and hold for 10 counts. Repeat to the other side.

Standing bow

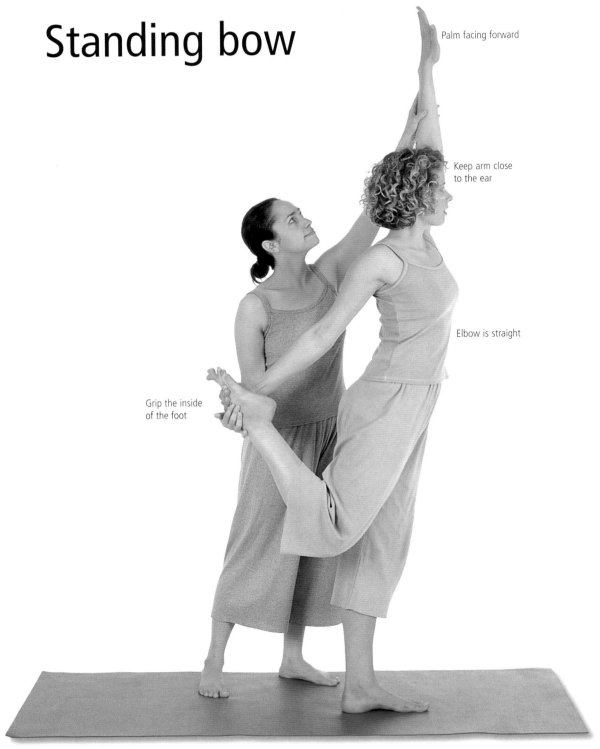

Palm facing forward

Keep arm close to the ear

Elbow is straight

Grip the inside of the foot

1 Stand tall with your feet together with arms at the side. Your partner should stand behind you. Take your right leg behind you and hold the inner side of the foot with your right hand. Take your left arm up close to the ear. Focus straight ahead. Your partner should help you steady your balance by holding your foot and arm. They should make sure you are in a straight line.

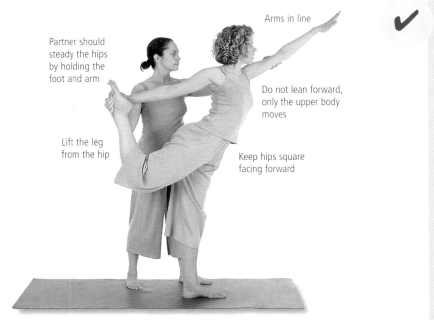

Partner should steady the hips by holding the foot and arm

Arms in line

Do not lean forward, only the upper body moves

Lift the leg from the hip

Keep hips square facing forward

2 Inhale, lift the right leg up from the hip as far as possible and then extend the left arm forward. Exhale, and breathe normally. Your partner should make sure that your shoulder is down and your elbow is straight.

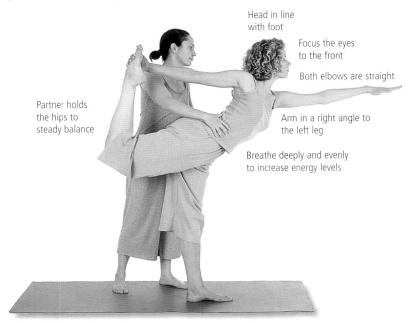

Head in line with foot

Focus the eyes to the front

Both elbows are straight

Partner holds the hips to steady balance

Arm in a right angle to the left leg

Breathe deeply and evenly to increase energy levels

3 Move your upper body smoothly, and balance on one leg. Create a beautiful arch with your spine. Keep stretching your back leg upward. Your partner should hold on to your waist to help you steady your balance and to make sure you are in a straight line. Imagine you are a dancer, and stretch forward and backward from your center. Hold for 30 counts. Repeat on the other side.

BENEFITS

This is called the Bow pose because of the beautiful arch of the spine. This stimulates the spine, improves circulation, and increases flexibility and energy levels. This is also called the dancer's pose, as it combines grace, beauty, poise, and balance. It is a physically demanding pose because you are combining strength, stamina, and intense concentration. The energy swirls around the body in a circular pattern, and you feel as light and fluid as air.

Physical
- Promotes youthfulness
- Tones legs, abdominal muscles
- Increases flexibility and suppleness of spine
- Increases energy levels
- Increases poise
- Promotes gracefulness
- Improves balance

Mental
- Improves concentration
- Focuses the mind
- Promotes mental balance
- Increases willpower

Health
- Improves circulation
- Prevents disease by unblocking energy centers
- Alleviates arthritis
- Helps sciatica and other back ailments

STANDING BOW

137

Wheel

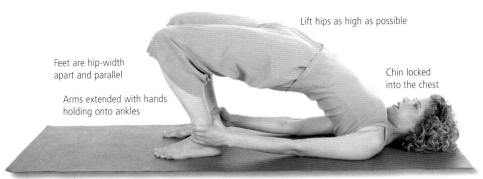

Lift hips as high as possible

Feet are hip-width apart and parallel

Arms extended with hands holding onto ankles

Chin locked into the chest

1 Lie flat, knees bent and in line with your hips and feet flat and as close to the buttocks as possible. Inhale and raise your buttocks as high as possible. Try to hold on to your ankles. Breathe normally. Lower down and repeat.

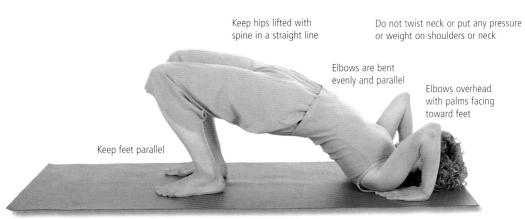

Keep hips lifted with spine in a straight line

Do not twist neck or put any pressure or weight on shoulders or neck

Elbows are bent evenly and parallel

Elbows overhead with palms facing toward feet

Keep feet parallel

2 Keeping your feet in the same position, lift your hips and buttocks and take your arms over your head with palms facing downward.

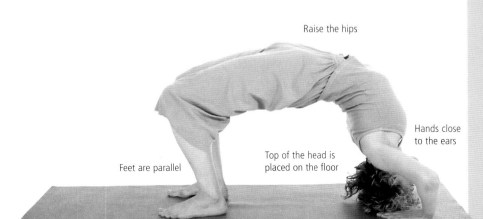

Raise the hips

Feet are parallel

Top of the head is placed on the floor

Hands close to the ears

3 Push up and rest on the crown of your head. Breathe normally and hold for 5–10 seconds.

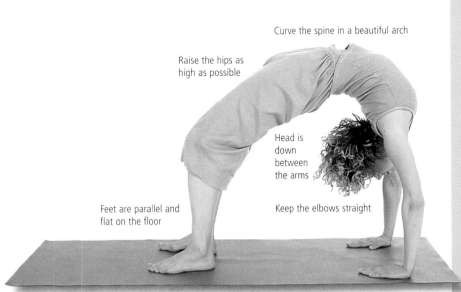

Curve the spine in a beautiful arch

Raise the hips as high as possible

Head is down between the arms

Feet are parallel and flat on the floor

Keep the elbows straight

4 Lift as high as possible, balancing on your toes and hands. Straighten your elbows and, breathing normally, hold for as long as possible. Return to Step 2, lift your head toward your chest and lower your spine, one vertebra at a time, with your tailbone last.

BENEFITS

This is an intense backbend, which stretches and invigorates the spine. It is physically challenging and builds muscles in the arms, tightens tummy and buttocks muscles, and tones the legs. It is an all-around exercise that keeps you fit from head to toe. Because of the position of the hands over the head, the heart rate increases, which burns calories. It also requires mental determination and stamina with strength and flexibility of the spine. Many people find this pose very difficult, but with continued practice, you will be able to master it.

Physical
- Tones the whole body, every muscle is working
- Flattens tummy
- Tightens buttocks muscles
- Strengthens the arms
- Increases suppleness of spine
- Tones legs
- Stretches neck

Mental
- Increases mental determination
- Increases self-confidence
- Increases willpower

Health
- Increases energy
- Unblocks stagnant energy fields
- Increases blood supply
- Stimulates heart rate
- Burns calories
- Regulates the thyroid
- Corrects hormone imbalance

Lying flat twist

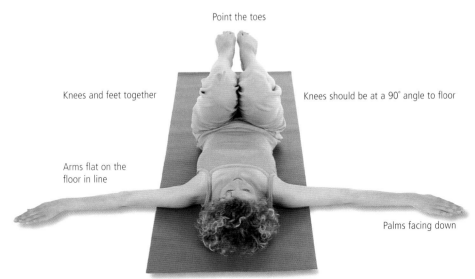

Point the toes

Knees and feet together

Knees should be at a 90° angle to floor

Arms flat on the floor in line

Palms facing down

1 Starting with Step 1 of Deep relaxation (see page 158), inhale and bring your knees toward the chest, keeping your lower legs parallel with the floor. Stretch your arms to the sides with palms face down. Look up, and relax the neck and shoulders. Keep your mouth closed and relax the jaw muscles.

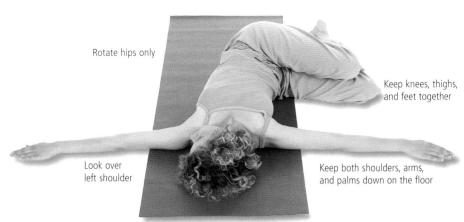

Rotate hips only

Keep knees, thighs, and feet together

Look over left shoulder

Keep both shoulders, arms, and palms down on the floor

2 Exhale, and bring both knees together down as close as possible to the right arm. Point your toes. Look to the left, and keep your shoulders down on the floor.

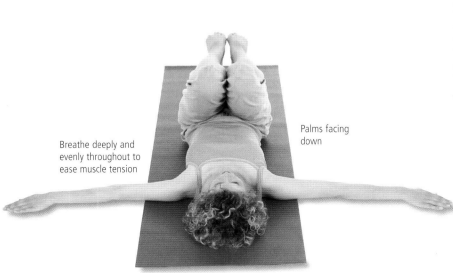

Breathe deeply and evenly throughout to ease muscle tension

Palms facing down

3 Inhale, and bring the head and knees back to center position. Keep the movement slow and smooth.

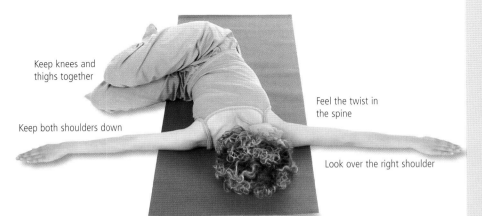

Keep knees and thighs together

Keep both shoulders down

Feel the twist in the spine

Look over the right shoulder

4 Exhale, and bring the knees over to the left. Look over to the right. Increase your stretch, and take your knees as close as possible to the left arm. Inhale, and return to Step 3. Repeat the whole exercise 4 times.

BENEFITS

This is a wonderful exercise to release back pain and tension in the neck, shoulders, upper, middle, and lower back. It is a gentle twist, and combined with deep breathing, relaxes the muscles and calms and soothes the nervous system. Many people when they suffer from back ailments believe they should move the spine as little as possible. Physicians now agree that it is important to first relieve the pain and then build the lower back muscles to prevent back pain from recurring. This exercise is often prescribed to achieve both.

Physical
• Has a feel-good factor
• Stretches entire spine
• Increases flexibility of the spine

Mental
• Soothes the nerves
• Promotes inner balance
• Improves mental stability

Health
• Alleviates back pain
• Prevents sciatica and lumbago
• Releases tension in upper body

Ayurvedic
• Good for all *doshas*, especially *Vata*

Rabbit

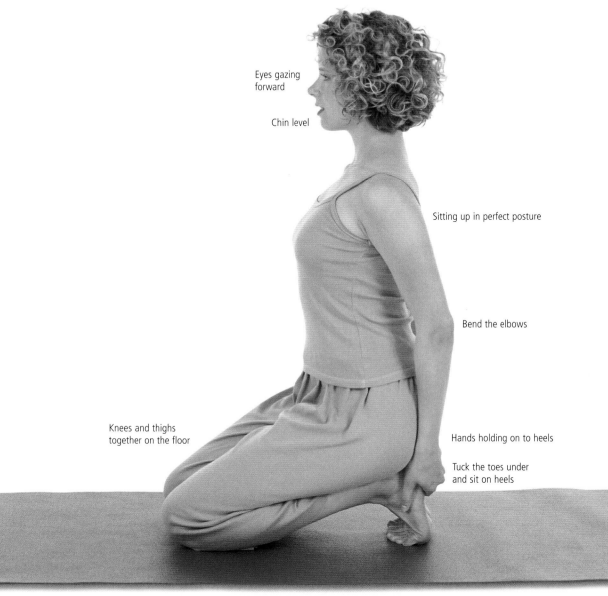

Eyes gazing forward

Chin level

Sitting up in perfect posture

Bend the elbows

Knees and thighs together on the floor

Hands holding on to heels

Tuck the toes under and sit on heels

1 Kneel on the floor, resting your buttocks on your heels, with your toes tucked under. Clasp your hands to your heels and sit up tall. Breathe normally.

BENEFITS

This pose is one of the most beneficial positions because it sends fresh oxygen into the brain, stimulating the spine and the entire nervous system. It helps prevent senility and promotes youthfulness and agility. In this position, the heartbeat slows down, and the brain, spine, and nerves receive a rich supply of nutrients.

Physical
- Has anti-aging effects
- Promotes a glowing complexion
- Promotes sparkling eyes

Mental
- Increases memory
- Improves concentration
- Increases ability to grasp intellectual thoughts
- Stimulates the senses
- Improves brain power
- Calms the nervous system

Health
- Helps prevent senility
- Has a beneficial effect on pituitary gland
- Balances thyroid
- Releases stress
- Relaxes the brain
- Strengthens the immune system

Ayurvedic
- Excellent for all *doshas*

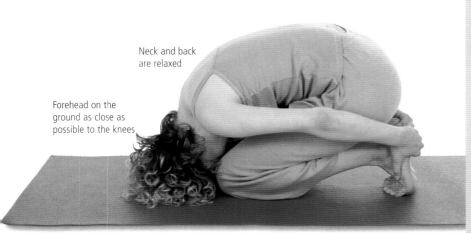

Neck and back are relaxed

Forehead on the ground as close as possible to the knees

2 Inhale, and as you exhale, curl your spine and place your forehead on the floor as close as you can to your knees. Breathe normally.

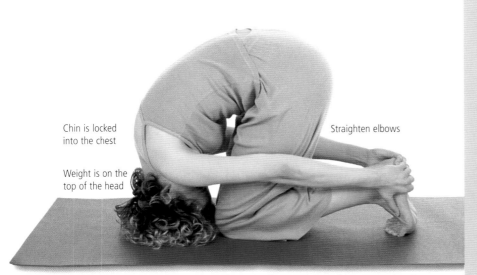

Chin is locked into the chest

Weight is on the top of the head

Straighten elbows

3 Roll on to the top of your head. Straighten your elbows and raise your hips. Breathe deeply and hold for 20 seconds. Return to Step 1 and repeat the exercise.

Dog

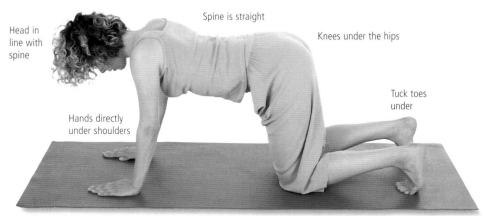

Head in line with spine

Spine is straight

Knees under the hips

Tuck toes under

Hands directly under shoulders

1 Kneel down on the floor, place the hands and arms directly under the shoulders and knees under the hips in a direct line. Keep the spine straight.

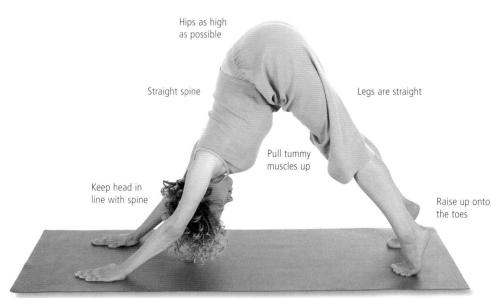

Hips as high as possible

Straight spine

Legs are straight

Pull tummy muscles up

Keep head in line with spine

Raise up onto the toes

2 Inhale, push the palms down to the floor, lift the body, and balance high onto the toes.

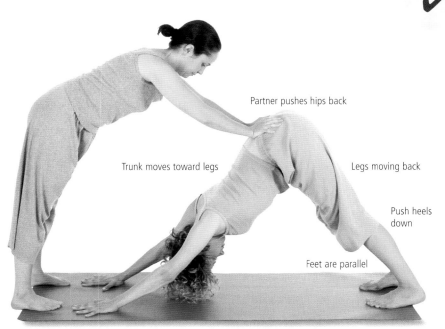

Partner pushes hips back

Trunk moves toward legs

Legs moving back

Push heels down

Feet are parallel

3 Exhale, breathe deeply and evenly. Grip the hands to the floor and push hips backward. Your partner should help you push your hips back by putting slight pressure onto the small of the back.

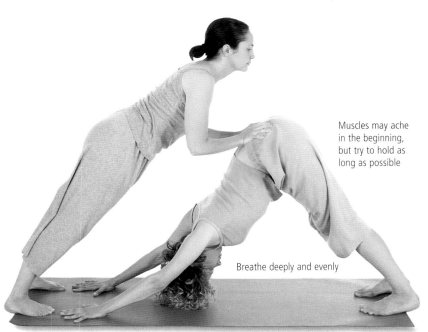

Muscles may ache in the beginning, but try to hold as long as possible

Breathe deeply and evenly

4 To increase the stretch, your partner should lean forward with their body weight in a straight line. Inhale and exhale, hold for as long as possible, or at least 30 counts. Distribute the weight evenly between your feet. Grip the floor hard with the feet and push the heels of your palms down to the floor and stretch the fingers out. Repeat.

BENEFITS

This pose strengthens and tones all the muscles in the physical body as well as calms the central nervous system. It is an intense stretch, and you can feel every muscle working from the toes all the way to the top of the head. The benefits of this exercise are felt when you are able to hold the position for a length of time. Stamina is increased and the immune system is boosted. As you hold the pose, breathe deeply, and push the heels down behind you, and draw the head toward the knees.

Physical
- Strengthens the body
- Increases stamina
- Tones the arms and legs
- Increases flexibility
- Increases energy

Mental
- Soothes the brain
- Promotes inner calm

Health
- Improves blood circulation
- Helps ease arthritis
- Balances hormones
- Aids lymph glands
- Increases energy flow to nervous system
- Keeps connective tissue healthy and pliable

Ayurvedic
- Especially good for *Pitta* and *Kapha* types

DOG

Spinal twist 2

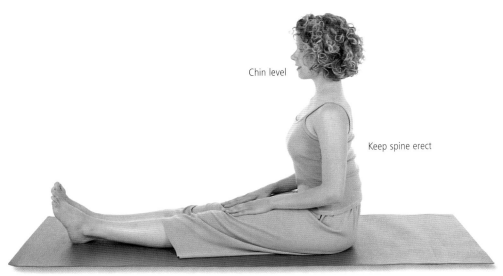

Chin level

Keep spine erect

1 Begin by sitting up tall with both legs stretched out in front of you and your hands resting gently on your thighs.

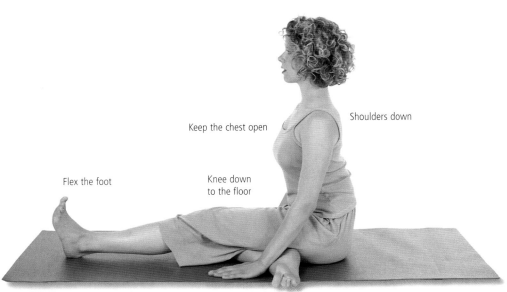

Keep the chest open

Shoulders down

Flex the foot

Knee down to the floor

2 Bring the right foot under the left thigh. Keep the right knee down by pushing the right hip downward. Place the right hand on the waist and left hand on the floor in front of your right foot.

BENEFITS

All spinal twists release tension and stress in the spine. Not only does it feel wonderful to twist from side to side, it also releases harmful toxins that build up in the body. Twists are an effective way to relieve headaches, backaches, and stiffness in the neck and shoulders. As you twist, the abdominal organs and kidneys are activated and exercised and the spine is energized and awakened. The spine becomes more supple and the mobility of the hips is increased.

Physical
- Increases flexibility
- Increases suppleness of the spine
- Promotes youthfulness
- Increases energy

Mental
- Calms the mind

Health
- Alleviates back pain
- Alleviates headaches
- Releases toxins
- Destresses nervous system
- Improves digestion
- Helps rheumatism
- Joints are lubricated
- Benefits gall bladder, liver, spleen, kidneys, and bowel
- Cures lethargy and sluggishness

Ayurvedic
- Good for *Vata* types

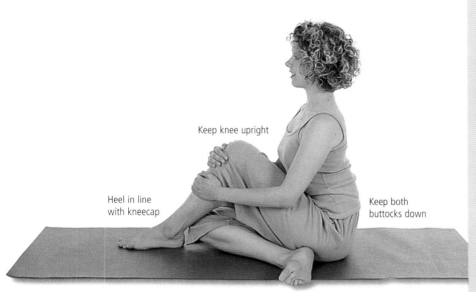

Keep knee upright

Heel in line with kneecap

Keep both buttocks down

3 Move the left leg farther under the right leg, making sure the kneecaps are in line with the hip bones. Keep the spine straight. Bend your right leg and bring your heel and ankle directly in front of the left knee in a straight line, with your hands on your right shin. Keep both buttocks down.

continued ▶

SPINAL TWIST 2

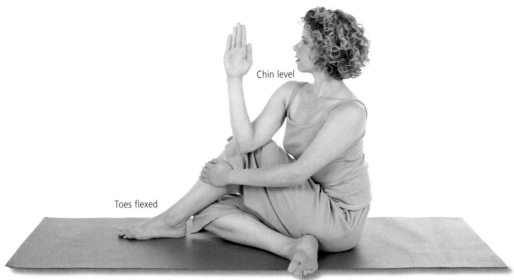

Chin level

Toes flexed

4 Rest your right elbow against the outside of your left knee and begin the twist around to your left. Exhale, breathe normally, and hold for 7 counts.

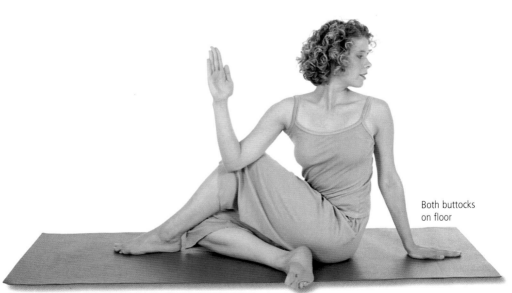

Both buttocks on floor

5 Place your left hand behind you, with the palm flat down on the floor and continue to twist round to the left. Exhale, breathe normally, and hold for 7 counts.

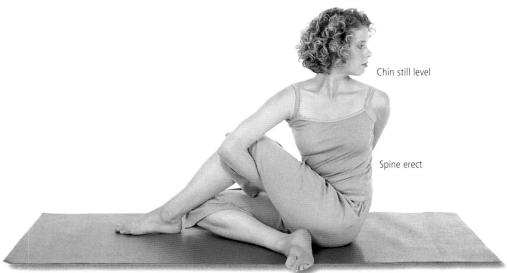

Chin still level

Spine erect

6 Link your hands under your left knee, keeping your spine erect and looking over your left shoulder. Exhale, breathe normally and hold for 7 counts. Return to Step 1 and repeat on the other side. Repeat the entire sequence 5 times.

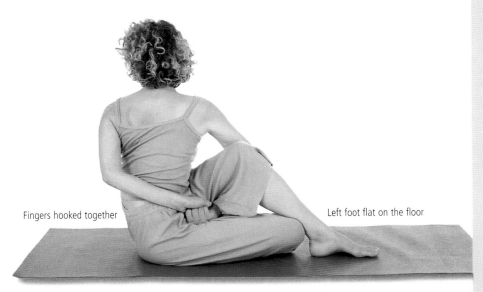

Fingers hooked together

Left foot flat on the floor

Step 6 viewed from the other side.

Spinal twist 3

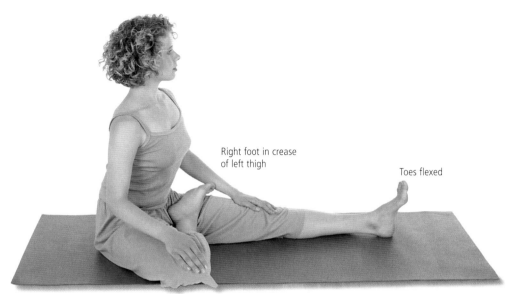

Right foot in crease
of left thigh

Toes flexed

1 Place your left leg directly in front of your hip and your right foot in the crease of your left thigh, keeping hips and thighs down. If you cannot reach this half lotus, place your right foot on your left thigh.

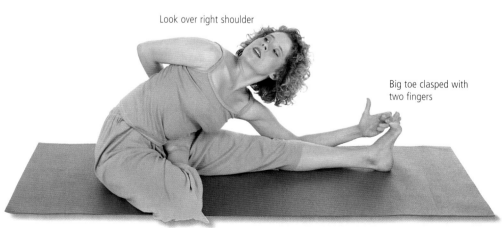

Look over right shoulder

Big toe clasped with
two fingers

2 Reach and clasp your left toes. Twist the spine and look over your right shoulder. Bring your right arm behind your back and clasp your right toes. Push thighs and knees down onto the floor and flex back your left big toe.

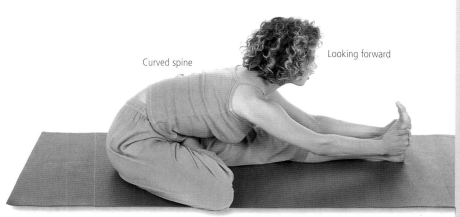

Curved spine

Looking forward

3 Release both arms and bring them forward. Stretch forward, elongating from the tailbone. Clasp fingertips around the back of the foot. If you cannot reach this far, place your hands on your knee or ankle.

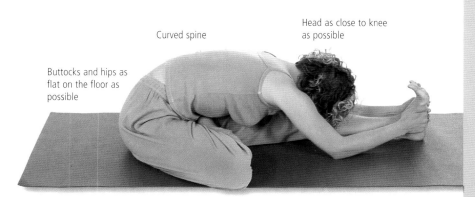

Curved spine

Head as close to knee as possible

Buttocks and hips as flat on the floor as possible

4 Relax farther forward, breathing deeply. Bring your head down as close as you can to your knee. Hold the position, then come up slowly.

BENEFITS

When the body is given a side twist, the spine becomes more supple. The muscles of the back are stimulated and the abdominal wall is toned. When the leg and foot are placed on the inner thigh in a half lotus position, tremendous pressure is placed on the liver and stomach, and some pressure is also placed on the kidneys and intestines. This means that all of the abdominal organs are massaged and circulation is increased, helping to eliminate poisons that are produced in the digestive process. Breathe normally throughout the sequence and hold each position for 5 seconds.

Physical
- Flattens tummy
- Increases suppleness
- Increases flexibility of the spine

Mental
- Soothes the brain
- Promotes clarity of thought

Health
- Destresses the nervous system

Breathe & relax 2

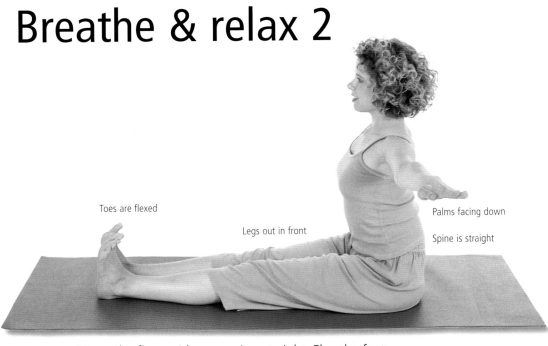

Toes are flexed

Legs out in front

Palms facing down

Spine is straight

1 Sit on the floor with your spine straight. Flex the feet with the toes pointing upward. Bring your arms out to the sides at shoulder height.

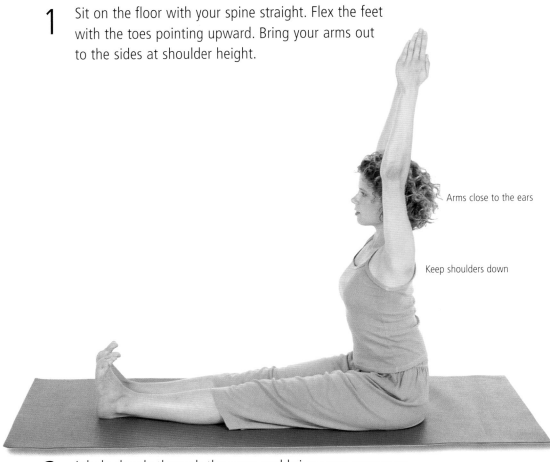

Arms close to the ears

Keep shoulders down

2 Inhale deeply through the nose and bring your arms over your head close to the ears.

BENEFITS

This exercise combines deep breathing with graceful movements that energize the spine and calm and soothe the brain. Deep breathing is a natural tranquilizer, which aids in blood circulation, lymph return, and energy flow to the nervous system. Most people only breathe one-third of their lung capacity and literally starve their bodies of valuable *prana,* or vital energy. This series is especially designed to help expand the chest and increase the oxygen levels in the body. This process feeds the brain and nourishes each cell. Without enough oxygen, metabolism cannot function and valuable nutrients, minerals, and vitamins are wasted. As you inhale, feel the lungs fill from the lower abdomen, expand into the ribcage or middle lungs, and upward into the top part of the lungs or chest. As you exhale fully, stale air, gaseous waste and toxins due to pollution are expelled.

Physical
- Increases energy levels
- Promotes glowing complexion
- Promotes sparkling eyes

Mental
- Promotes inner calm
- Soothes the brain
- Promotes inner peace
- Promotes mental balance and harmony

Health
- Counteracts pollution
- Improves circulation
- Builds immune system
- Combats stress
- Helps prevent illness and diseases

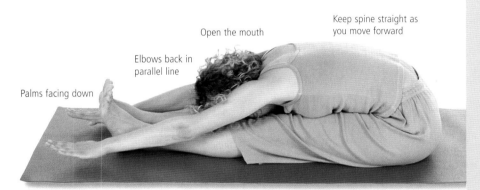

Palms facing down

Elbows back in parallel line

Open the mouth

Keep spine straight as you move forward

3 Open the mouth, exhale, and blow the air out as you move your body forward over your legs. Bring your arms close to the head with palms facing down. Relax the spine over the body. Relax the feet, legs, and arms. Inhale and exhale, and hold for 10–15 counts.

Rejuvenation

Rejuvenation is one of the key goals for people who practice yoga to maintain youth and vitality. The mental attitude is as important as the dexterity and flexibility of the spine, and when you feel youthful, you glow with well-being. The secret of rejuvenation is the combination of stretching with *Pranayama*, or breathing techniques. Always concentrate on the breathing and feel the lungs fill to their full capacity. This strengthens the diaphragm and increases fresh oxygen to the entire system.

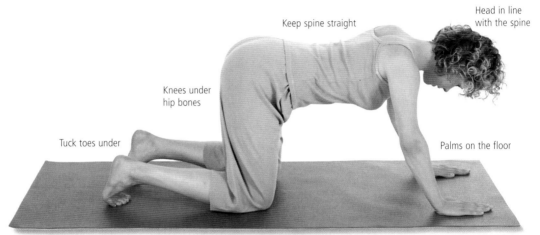

Keep spine straight

Head in line
with the spine

Knees under
hip bones

Tuck toes under

Palms on the floor

1 Kneel on the floor. Place your knees under your hip bones and tuck your toes under. Keep your spine straight and place your palms under your shoulder blades. Keep your head in line with your spine.

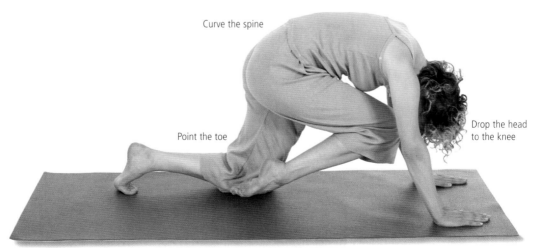

Curve the spine

Point the toe

Drop the head
to the knee

2 Inhale deeply, drop your head down, and bring your right knee up toward your forehead.

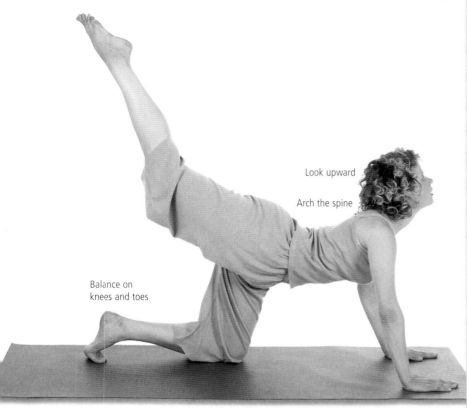

Look upward

Arch the spine

Balance on
knees and toes

3 Exhale deeply and slowly, arch your spine like a cat, and lift the leg up as high as possible behind you. Keep the hips square and point the toe. Look upward to increase the stretch.

Knee is on the floor

Chest rests on the knee

Drop forehead
down to the floor

Leg is straight
behind you

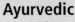

Point the toe

4 Inhale, and as you exhale, slowly lower the leg down to the floor. Relax the spine and drop the forehead down to the floor to relax the brain. Stretch the arms out in front of you. Inhale and exhale and hold for at least 10 counts. Repeat on the other side and continue the sequence 5 times on each side to reap the benefits.

BENEFITS

This exercise improves circulation and increases suppleness of the spine. The stretch combined with deep and deliberate breath control unblocks energy that is trapped in the 7 *chakras* of the spine. It increases vitality and energy levels and physically enhances the complexion, giving a youthful appearance. The entire back is toned and all the stress and tension in the spine is released. Synchronize the breath with the movements and stretch the leg up and back as high as you can keeping the hips in line.

Physical
- Increases suppleness
- Increases flexibility of the spine
- Tones the legs
- Tightens buttock muscles
- Strengthens the arms

Mental
- Soothes the brain
- Increases concentration
- Promotes gracefulness
- Promotes positive thinking

Health
- Improves circulation
- Cures fatigue
- Boosts energy levels
- Releases toxins

Ayurvedic
- Good for *Kapha* types

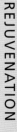

REJUVENATION

Nerve soother

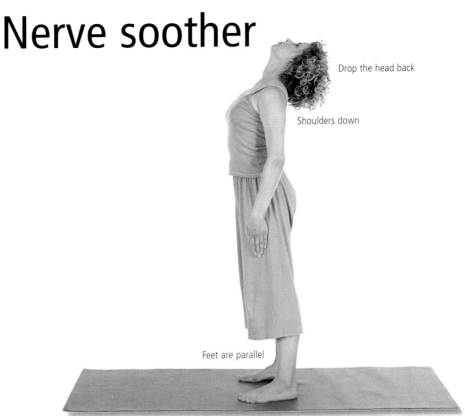

Drop the head back

Shoulders down

Feet are parallel

1 Stand tall in perfect posture with your feet at hip width. Place your arms at your sides. Inhale deeply and drop your head back, keeping your shoulders down.

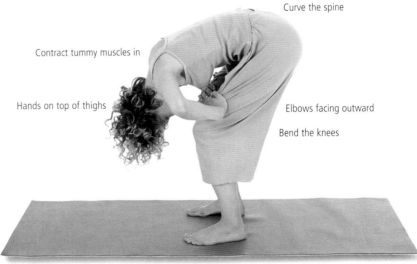

Curve the spine

Contract tummy muscles in

Hands on top of thighs

Elbows facing outward

Bend the knees

2 Open your mouth, exhale, and blow vigorously through the mouth as if you are blowing out a candle until all the breath is out of the lungs. Contract the body forward, bend the knees, and place your hands on the top of your thighs.

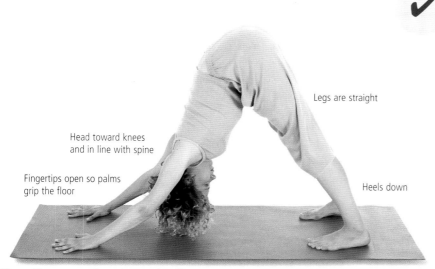

Legs are straight

Head toward knees
and in line with spine

Fingertips open so palms
grip the floor

Heels down

3 Place your hands on the floor. Move your feet back to create a V-shape with your spine. Keep the heels down and bring the head back toward the knees to increase the stretch. Keep the spine straight. Breathe normally and deeply, and hold for 10 counts.

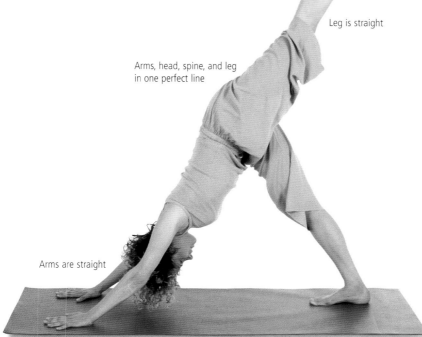

Point the toe

Leg is straight

Arms, head, spine, and leg
in one perfect line

Arms are straight

4 Inhale, raise the left leg as high as possible, keeping the leg in line with the spine. Point the toe. Exhale, breathe normally for 10 counts. Repeat on the other side and repeat the whole sequence twice more.

BENEFITS

Breathing from the diaphragm acts as a natural tranquilizer to the nervous system. The deeper you breathe, the calmer the mind becomes. You don't even need to believe in it because it is a natural process. As you inhale, concentrate on the mental and physical stress you feel in the mind and body and as you exhale, release all negative thoughts and emotions. It is important to learn to regulate your breathing pattern to reduce stress at a deeper level. Many people, when they are stressed, quicken the breath and actually reduce their oxygen intake, which can lead to hypertension and panic attacks As you practice yoga breathing techniques, you will find inner peace and find a sense of inner calm.

Physical
- Relaxes the face
- Releases tension in neck and shoulders
- Stretches neck
- Increases circulation to face

Mental
- Promotes tranquility
- Promotes inner calm
- Soothes the nerves
- Calms the brain
- Releases negative thoughts and emotions

Health
- Cures respiratory disorders such as bronchitis
- Helps asthma
- Prevents hypertension
- Avoids panic attack
- Reduces stress on all levels

NERVE SOOTHER

157

Deep relaxation

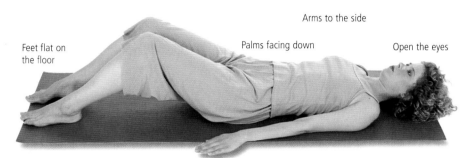

Feet flat on
the floor

Palms facing down

Arms to the side

Open the eyes

1 Lie down flat and bring your knees up with feet flat on the floor.
Place your arms at your sides in line with the shoulders, with the
palms facing down.

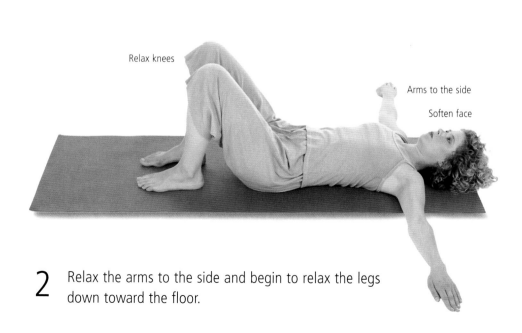

Relax knees

Arms to the side

Soften face

2 Relax the arms to the side and begin to relax the legs
down toward the floor.

BENEFITS

Learning the art of relaxation is an invaluable technique that teaches you how to turn your attention inward and control with visualization every aspect of your mind and body. This works on the deeper levels of the mental, physical, and emotional layers to reduce stress and promote well-being. This exercise rejuvenates and recharges valuable energy, or *prana*, lost through mental and physical imbalance. Complete tranquility allows the body to restore the equilibrium and find peace of mind.

Physical
- Increases body's energy levels
- Relaxes muscles
- Increases energy

Mental
- Releases mental fatigue
- Calms and soothes nerves
- Boosts brainpower
- Clarifies thoughts
- Crystallizes future
- Balances mental, physical, and spiritual
- Promotes stillness of the mind
- Improves mind control

Health
- Cures nervous disorders
- Cures insomnia
- Provides understanding of mental health
- Increases power of mind over negative thoughts and emotions
- Helps prevent diseases
- Rebalances energy
- Rejuvenates internal organs

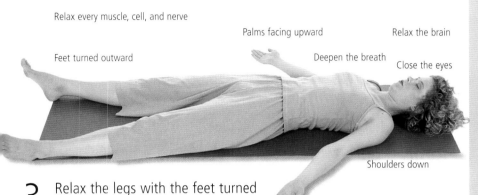

Relax every muscle, cell, and nerve

Palms facing upward

Relax the brain

Feet turned outward

Deepen the breath

Close the eyes

Shoulders down

3 Relax the legs with the feet turned outward. Face palms upward. Relax all the muscles in the face and body. Breathe deeply and evenly for 10 counts. Isolate each muscle group, starting from the feet up toward the head by tensing and releasing. Relax the brain. Concentrate only on the breath. 15 minutes of deep relaxation is equal to 5 hours of deep sleep.

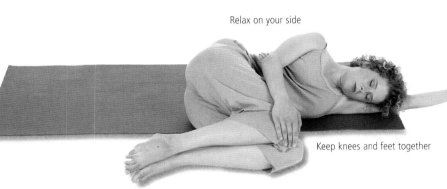

Relax on your side

Keep knees and feet together

4 To release, bring both knees into the chest, and roll over to the side. Relax as long as you wish before getting up, or you can use this technique before bedtime to help you sleep.

yoga for the mind & spirit

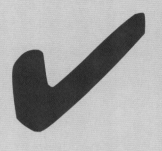

Kalaripayatt is believed to be the oldest and most comprehensive system of martial arts. Its roots originate from the twelfth century and it forms a part of the Indian sciences that include *Ayurveda* and yoga. It is known as a martial/healing arts system that combines beautiful yet dynamic and powerful forms of yoga based exercises and meditation.

Kalari is where the training begins and it is known as "the temple of learning." It is here that religious and spiritual lessons begin along with the learning of total control over mind and body. Every movement begins and ends with the breath to achieve stillness at the very core of one's center, which allows the body to "become all eyes." Physical strength, endurance, and quickness of the mind are essential for combat, and the practice of yoga creates greater suppleness while focusing the mind.

Learning yoga and *Pranayama* (breathing techniques) sharpens and steadies the mind and gives courage and patience with a fighting spirit. It unlocks the body's natural flow of internal energy to create a total Martial Arts/Meditation system of movement.

Breath control

Pranayama is the science of breath control. A yogi's life is not measured by days but by the number of breaths. The rhythmic patterns of slow, deep breathing strengthen the respiratory system, soothe the nervous system, and reduce cravings. When desires and cravings are diminished, the mind is set free and becomes a vehicle for concentration. Through learning the deep, steady meaning of inhalation and exhalation, the mind is trained to become still.

When the mind is emptied of useless thoughts and emotions, one can focus on a single thought and find inner peace. To stop the mind from wandering is the essence of meditation. This enables one to control the senses and reach the final stage of enlightenment. It is said that the mind is pure and impure. It is pure when it is free from desires, and impure when it thrives on desire.

How does meditation work?

Meditation rids impurity and focuses on joining the pure power of the cosmic universe to achieve spiritual bliss. It teaches us to go deeper into our darkest realms to reach for salvation. Every question and every answer lie within us, and yoga teaches us how to tap into the great knowledge and find spirituality, not based on religious beliefs but on universal truths. It is a great gift to become connected to our higher consciousness and intuition. It gives us a power to control our own destiny and spiritual progress. Yoga meditation is an invaluable tool to master the mind and spirit.

Meditation in motion

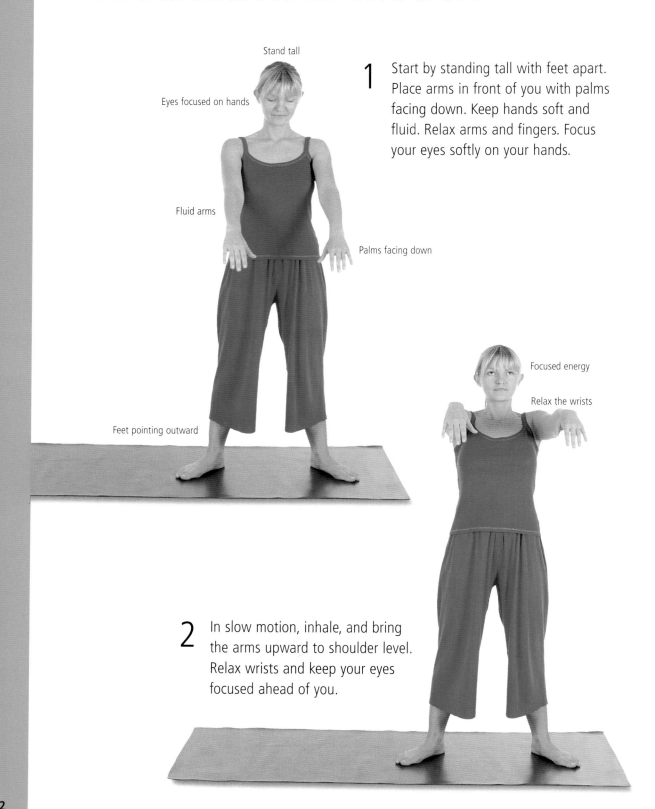

Stand tall

Eyes focused on hands

Fluid arms

Palms facing down

Feet pointing outward

1 Start by standing tall with feet apart. Place arms in front of you with palms facing down. Keep hands soft and fluid. Relax arms and fingers. Focus your eyes softly on your hands.

Focused energy

Relax the wrists

2 In slow motion, inhale, and bring the arms upward to shoulder level. Relax wrists and keep your eyes focused ahead of you.

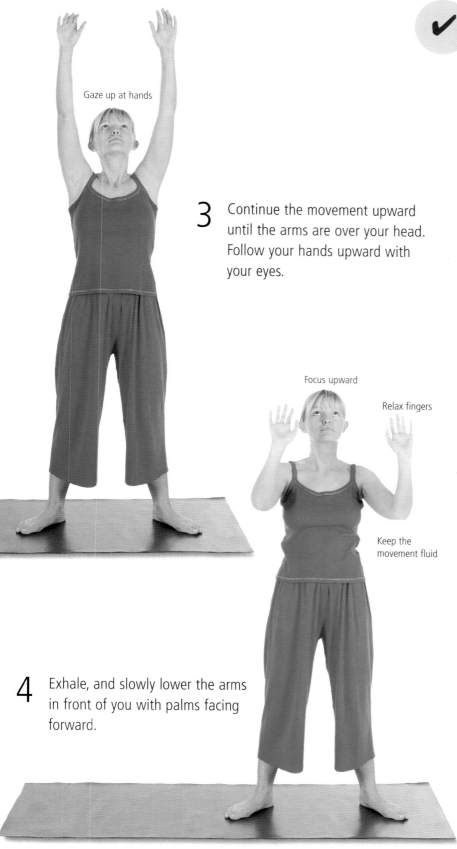

Gaze up at hands

3 Continue the movement upward until the arms are over your head. Follow your hands upward with your eyes.

Focus upward

Relax fingers

Keep the movement fluid

4 Exhale, and slowly lower the arms in front of you with palms facing forward.

BENEFITS

This series of flowing movements begins to help you understand how to turn your attention inward. By moving slowly with a great awareness of the breath, the mind starts to quiet down and become almost still. It is an excellent way to push out bothersome and troubling thoughts to concentrate only on the movement itself. It trains the mind and body to work in unison, which improves coordination and clarity of thought. The emphasis should be on keeping the pace even. Imagine that you are a dancer and that you are moving in slow motion from one position to another.

Physical
- Improves physical coordination
- Improves balance
- Improves poise
- Improves fitness level
- Increases energy

Mental
- Improves ental concentration
- Promotes positive thinking
- Promotes clarity of thoughts
- Focuses the mind

Health
- Improves circulation
- Calms the brain
- Increases oxygen to the blood

Ayurvedic
- Excellent for all *doshas*

continued ▶

MEDITATION IN MOTION

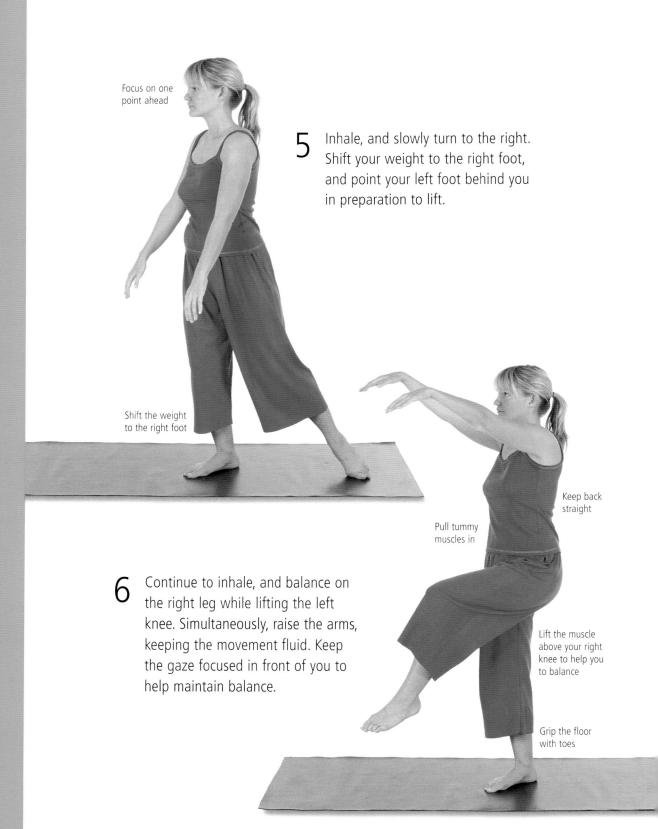

Focus on one
point ahead

5 Inhale, and slowly turn to the right.
Shift your weight to the right foot,
and point your left foot behind you
in preparation to lift.

Shift the weight
to the right foot

Keep back
straight

Pull tummy
muscles in

6 Continue to inhale, and balance on
the right leg while lifting the left
knee. Simultaneously, raise the arms,
keeping the movement fluid. Keep
the gaze focused in front of you to
help maintain balance.

Lift the muscle
above your right
knee to help you
to balance

Grip the floor
with toes

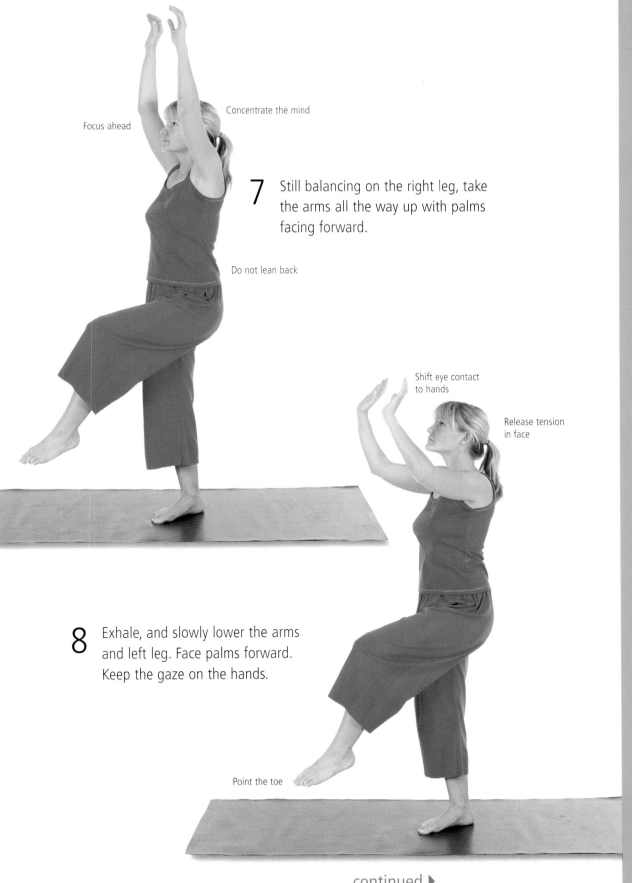

Focus ahead

Concentrate the mind

7 Still balancing on the right leg, take the arms all the way up with palms facing forward.

Do not lean back

Shift eye contact to hands

Release tension in face

8 Exhale, and slowly lower the arms and left leg. Face palms forward. Keep the gaze on the hands.

Point the toe

continued ▶

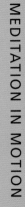

MEDITATION IN MOTION

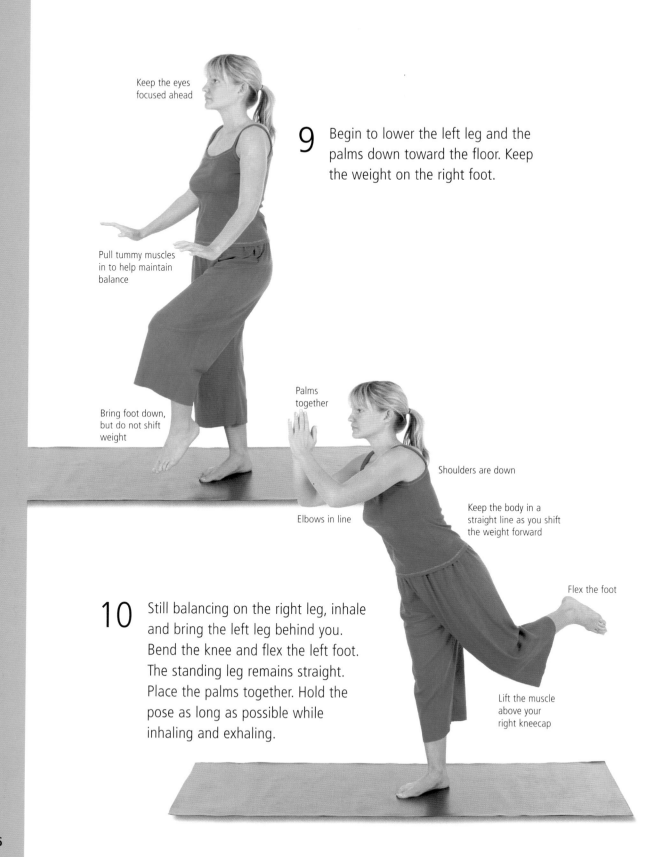

Keep the eyes focused ahead

9 Begin to lower the left leg and the palms down toward the floor. Keep the weight on the right foot.

Pull tummy muscles in to help maintain balance

Bring foot down, but do not shift weight

Palms together

Shoulders are down

Elbows in line

Keep the body in a straight line as you shift the weight forward

Flex the foot

10 Still balancing on the right leg, inhale and bring the left leg behind you. Bend the knee and flex the left foot. The standing leg remains straight. Place the palms together. Hold the pose as long as possible while inhaling and exhaling.

Lift the muscle above your right kneecap

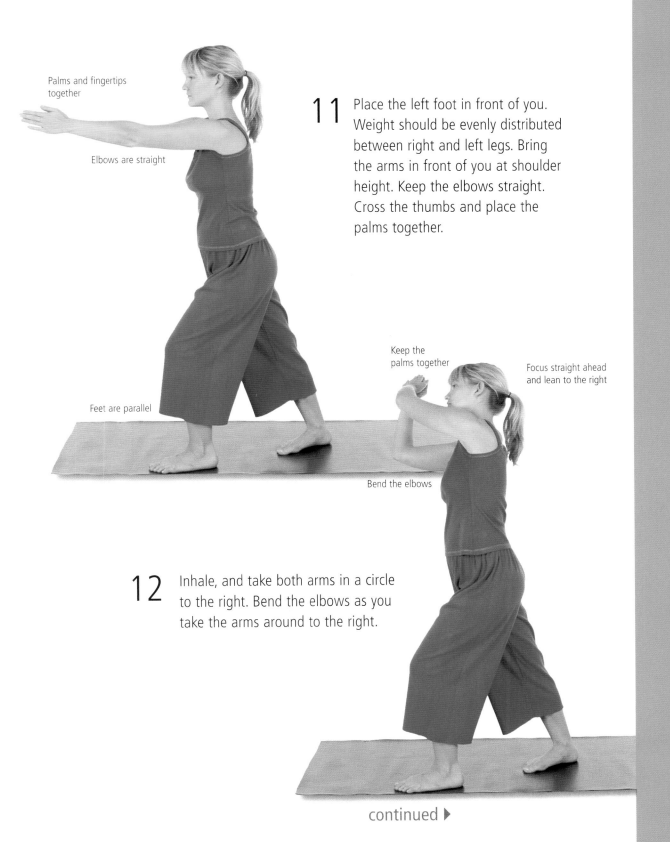

Palms and fingertips together

Elbows are straight

Feet are parallel

11 Place the left foot in front of you. Weight should be evenly distributed between right and left legs. Bring the arms in front of you at shoulder height. Keep the elbows straight. Cross the thumbs and place the palms together.

Keep the palms together

Focus straight ahead and lean to the right

Bend the elbows

12 Inhale, and take both arms in a circle to the right. Bend the elbows as you take the arms around to the right.

continued ▶

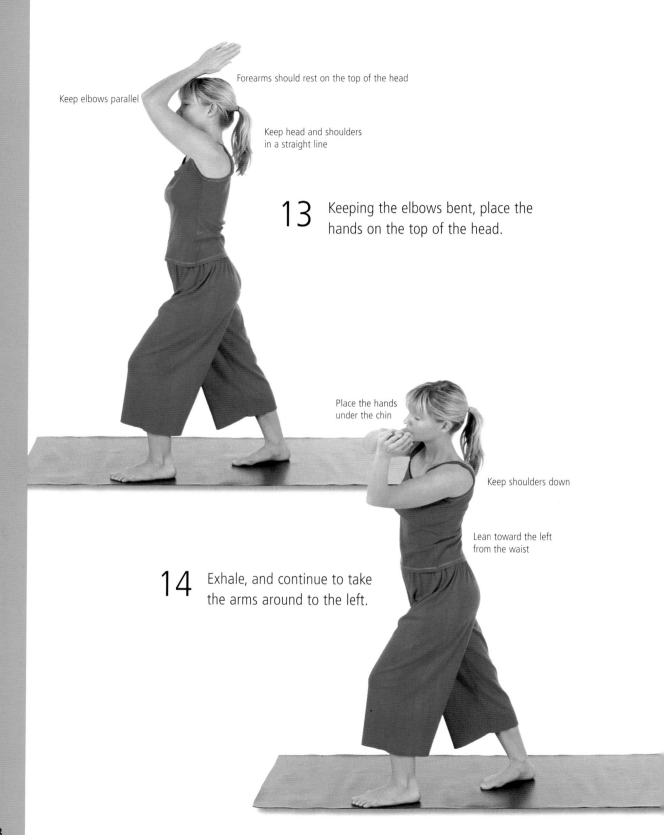

Forearms should rest on the top of the head

Keep elbows parallel

Keep head and shoulders in a straight line

13 Keeping the elbows bent, place the hands on the top of the head.

Place the hands under the chin

Keep shoulders down

Lean toward the left from the waist

14 Exhale, and continue to take the arms around to the left.

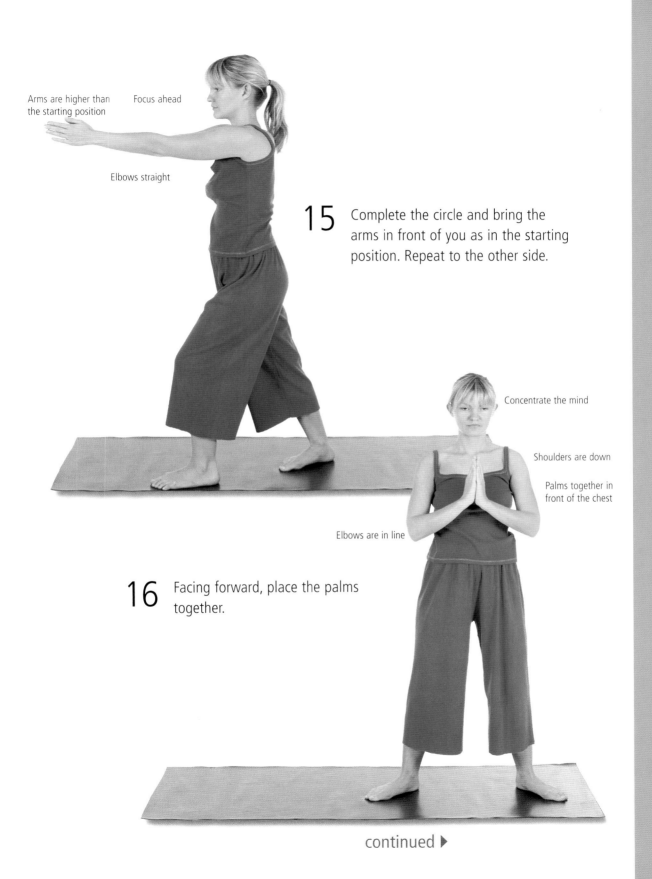

Arms are higher than the starting position

Focus ahead

Elbows straight

15 Complete the circle and bring the arms in front of you as in the starting position. Repeat to the other side.

Concentrate the mind

Shoulders are down

Palms together in front of the chest

Elbows are in line

16 Facing forward, place the palms together.

continued ▶

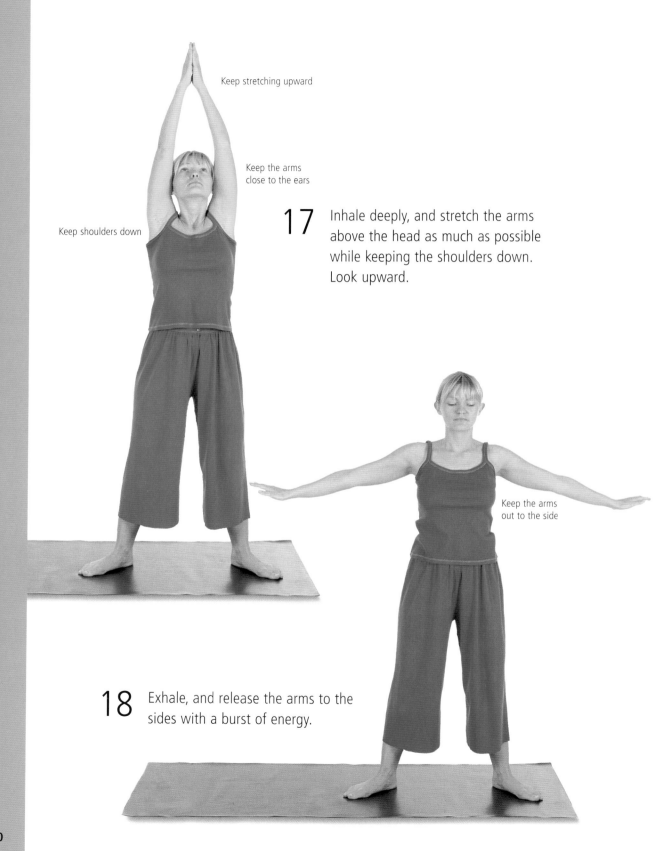

Keep stretching upward

Keep the arms
close to the ears

Keep shoulders down

17 Inhale deeply, and stretch the arms above the head as much as possible while keeping the shoulders down. Look upward.

Keep the arms
out to the side

18 Exhale, and release the arms to the sides with a burst of energy.

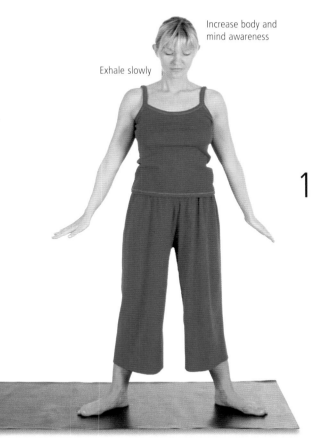

Exhale slowly

Increase body and mind awareness

19   Still exhaling, lower the arms with palms facing downward.

20   Relax the arms to the sides. Keep the eyes gazing downward. Inhale and exhale, and hold for 5 counts. Still exhaling, lower the left leg and both arms.

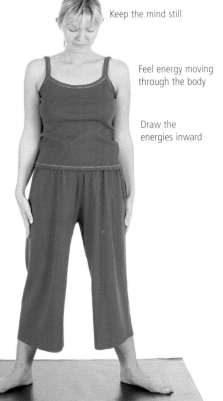

Keep the mind still

Feel energy moving through the body

Draw the energies inward

Horse

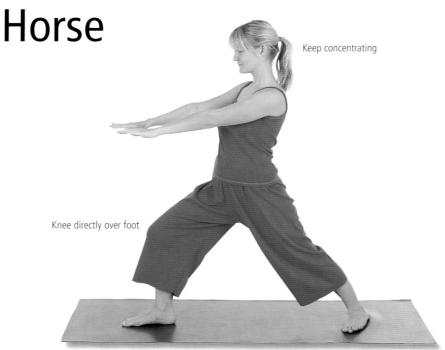

Keep concentrating

Knee directly over foot

1 Stand with your legs hip-width apart and your arms raised parallel in front of you. Keeping your mind focused, swing yourself purposefully but gracefully to the right, allowing your feet to rotate slightly.

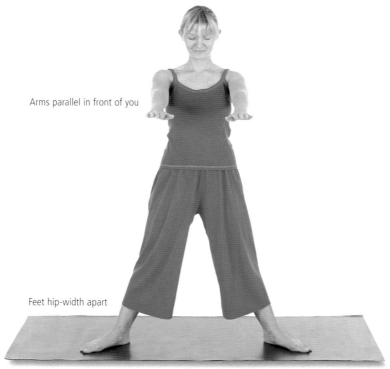

Arms parallel in front of you

Feet hip-width apart

2 Return to your starting position, keeping your eyes lowered.

BENEFITS

The initiation of the warrior begins with animal poses that are associated with combat. The Horse traditionally is trained by the horseman to be swift and steady. This exercise teaches you the art of focusing the mind, while the body moves from one direction to the next. The philosophy states that one should never lose sight of one's opponent. This exercise clearly helps to train the mind to concentrate while developing a fighting spirit. Remember to move smoothly and gracefully while maintaining power and strength.

Physical
- Improves poise and grace
- Improves balance
- Trims waist
- Tones legs

Mental
- Improves concentration
- Trains the mind to focus
- Improves memory
- Increases courage
- Promotes positive thinking

Allow the feet to rotate slightly

3 Repeat the swing to the other side, maintaining your concentration. Repeat the whole sequence 5–7 times.

Ayurvedic
- Good for *Vata* types

HORSE

Elephant

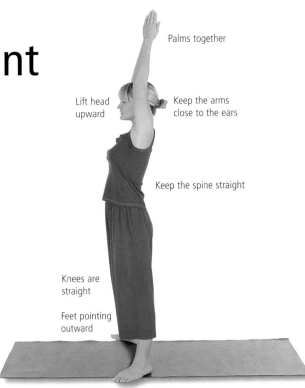

Palms together

Lift head upward

Keep the arms close to the ears

Keep the spine straight

Knees are straight

Feet pointing outward

1 Stand with your feet in a wide second position with toes pointing outward. Stand tall and take your arms over your head stretching upward. Cross the thumbs and keep the palms and fingers together, as in a prayer pose. Keep the gaze straight ahead. Inhale and exhale.

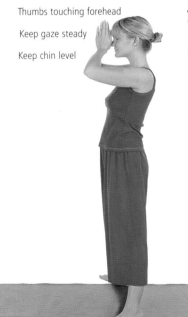

Thumbs touching forehead

Keep gaze steady

Keep chin level

2 Inhale, and bring your palms in front of your face. The thumbs should rest on the forehead. Keep the head upright, and focus on the hands. Keep elbows in line with shoulders.

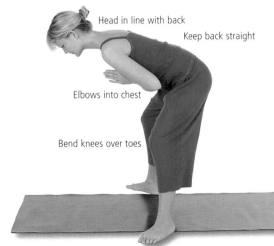

Head in line with back

Keep back straight

Elbows into chest

Bend knees over toes

3 Continue to inhale, bend the knees, and move the body forward while keeping the back straight. Bring the elbows together toward the chest.

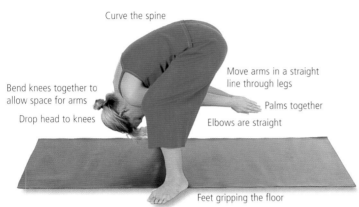

Curve the spine

Bend knees together to allow space for arms

Drop head to knees

Move arms in a straight line through legs

Palms together

Elbows are straight

Feet gripping the floor

4 In a swift movement, drop the head to the knees, and move the arms through the legs to the back. Keep the arms straight and palms together.

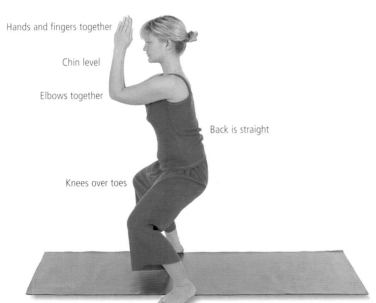

Hands and fingers together

Chin level

Elbows together

Back is straight

Knees over toes

5 Exhale, and take the back upright while keeping the knees bent. Keep the elbows together with the hands in front of the forehead. Keep the gaze to the hands. Inhale and exhale. Continue to hold for 10 counts. Repeat 5 times.

BENEFITS

The elephant is the animal of strength and power. This exercise improves physical strength, and the wide stance empowers and steadies the mind. *Kalari* teaches that 80 percent of physical power is in the mind so when you perform the final pose, feel the power and strength of your mind and body. Before you begin, imagine the courage and patience that you need to defend yourself against a deadly foe.

Physical
- Strengthens the entire body
- Tones the legs
- Improves stamina
- Increases flexibly
- Increases suppleness of the spine
- Promotes dynamic energy

Mental
- Increases alertness
- Increases awareness
- Promotes positive thinking
- Increases power
- Increases courage

Health
- Increases circulation
- Improves breath control
- Increases oxygen to blood supply
- Stimulates brain function

Ayurvedic
- Good for *Pitta* types

ELEPHANT

Lion

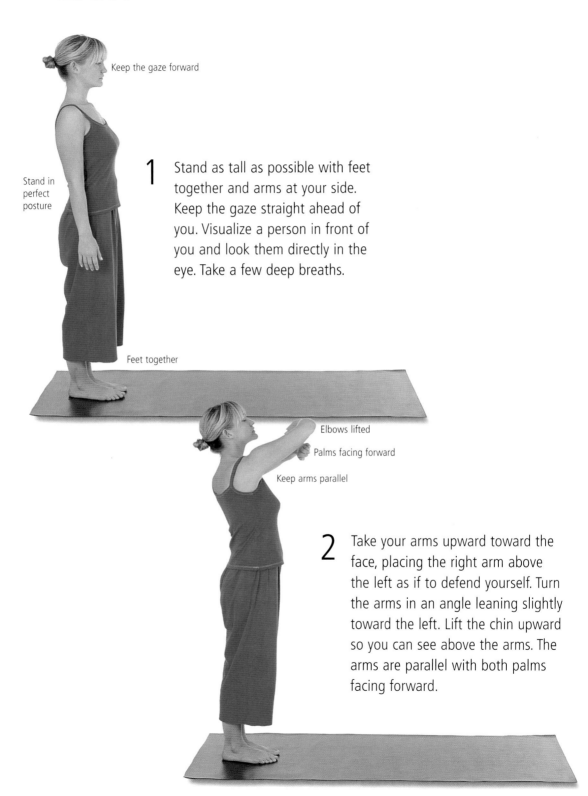

Keep the gaze forward

Stand in perfect posture

1 Stand as tall as possible with feet together and arms at your side. Keep the gaze straight ahead of you. Visualize a person in front of you and look them directly in the eye. Take a few deep breaths.

Feet together

Elbows lifted

Palms facing forward

Keep arms parallel

2 Take your arms upward toward the face, placing the right arm above the left as if to defend yourself. Turn the arms in an angle leaning slightly toward the left. Lift the chin upward so you can see above the arms. The arms are parallel with both palms facing forward.

BENEFITS

The lion epitomizes agility, skillfulness, power, and, above all, courage. It is a training exercise that teaches you how to move through space with coordinated movements, never letting go of eye contact with the person who is directly in front of you. After learning the movement for yourself, practice with a partner so as you move forward they will be moving backward. Then change direction and move the other way. It is important to be intimidating and forceful by using eye contact with fluid movement. The idea is that if you were using weapons in battle with an adversary, they cannot anticipate your next move. With the dexterity and sharpness of the mind, any battle can be fought and won.

Physical
- Increases strength
- Improves stamina
- Increases energy levels
- Increases quickness of movement
- Increases coordination

Mental
- Increases quickness of mind
- Increases alertness
- Promotes clarity of mind
- Enhances steadfastness of mind
- Promotes positive thinking
- Empowers

Health
- Increases mind and body awareness
- Builds immune system
- Improves circulation
- Burns calories

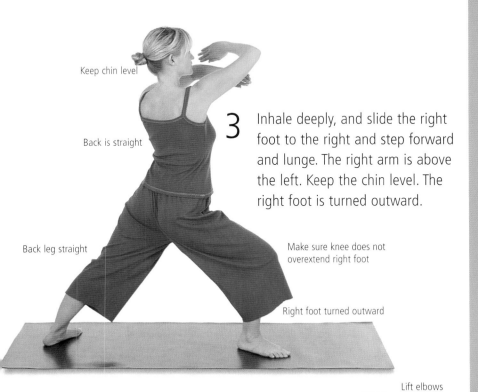

Keep chin level

Back is straight

Back leg straight

3 Inhale deeply, and slide the right foot to the right and step forward and lunge. The right arm is above the left. Keep the chin level. The right foot is turned outward.

Make sure knee does not overextend right foot

Right foot turned outward

Lift elbows

Keep the gaze straight ahead

Keep shoulders down

Slightly tilt torso to the right

4 Moving forward, step out to the left with the left foot and change arms so that the left arm is above the right. Keep the momentum moving forward as you slide your feet. Reverse and move backward. Repeat 5 times forward and backward.

Left foot turned outward

Leg kicks

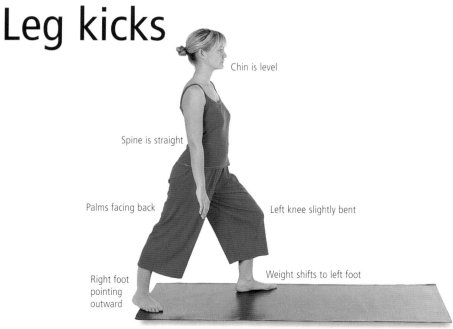

Chin is level

Spine is straight

Palms facing back

Left knee slightly bent

Right foot pointing outward

Weight shifts to left foot

1 Stand tall with feet together and arms at your side. Step back with the right foot in preparation for the kick. Keep spine upright and focus the eyes straight ahead on one spot.

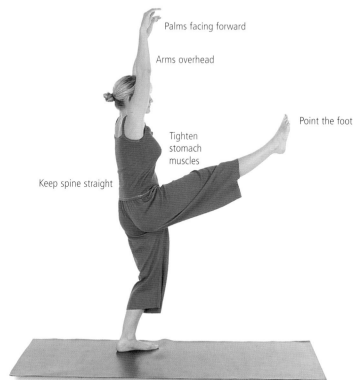

Palms facing forward

Arms overhead

Point the foot

Tighten stomach muscles

Keep spine straight

2 Inhale, and kick the right leg upward as high as possible without collapsing the spine. Simultaneously, lift the arms over the head and bend left knee slightly.

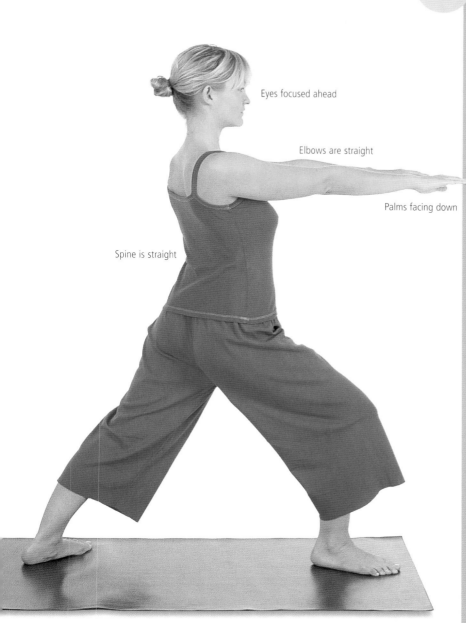

Eyes focused ahead

Elbows are straight

Palms facing down

Spine is straight

3 Exhale, and step forward onto right foot. Keep the right knee bent in preparation to kick with the opposite leg. Keep elbows straight, with arms in front at shoulder height. Your palms should be facing downward. Repeat on the opposite side and do 5 to 6 sets in one direction, and then reverse and do the same number the other way.

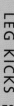

BENEFITS

These leg kicks increase the flexibility of the body and awaken the mind to act swiftly and precisely. Even though it is an easy movement, it still combines balance and coordination with mind control. Keep the kicks steady and even. Do not worry about the height of the kick. The back should remain upright throughout. Avoid the tendency to collapse the spine while raising the leg. Move forward through space and do at least 5 to 6 kicks forward to experience the element of combat. After finishing the set, turn around and move in the opposite direction. Repeat 3 times in both directions.

Physical
- Strengthens the legs
- Tones legs and abdominal muscles
- Improves balance and coordination
- Increases poise

Mental
- Focuses the mind
- Promotes positive thinking
- Empowers
- Increases discipline

Health
- Improves circulation
- Adds fresh oxygen to blood supply
- Keeps connective tissue healthy and pliable

Circles

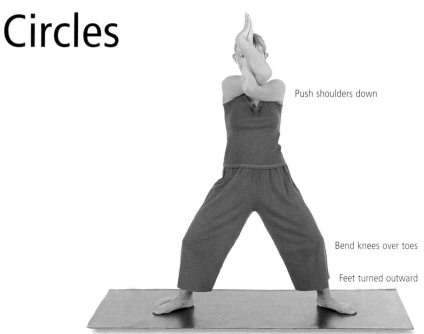

Push shoulders down

Bend knees over toes

Feet turned outward

1 Stand with your feet wide apart and turned outward. Bring your arms out to the sides in line with the shoulders. Bring the right arm under the left, crossing them at the elbows, keeping both shoulders down. Twist your right hand toward your left palm in front of your nose, and press the palms together. Push the shoulder blades down. Bend both knees over the toes.

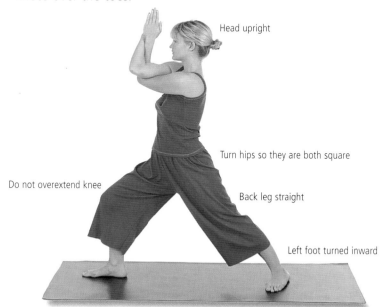

Head upright

Turn hips so they are both square

Do not overextend knee

Back leg straight

Left foot turned inward

2 Holding the arm position, turn the right foot to the right and lunge to the right. You are facing exactly sideways. Keep the eyes focused ahead and make sure the knee does not overextend the right foot. The right heel should be in line with the instep of the left foot.

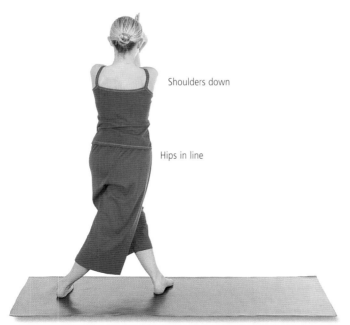

Shoulders down

Hips in line

3 Keeping the body in a straight line, keep turning the body to the right and cross the left leg in front of the right so you are facing the opposite direction from when you started the exercise.

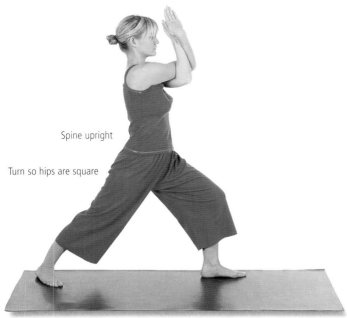

Spine upright

Turn so hips are square

4 Keep turning to the right until you are facing exactly sideways and lunge with your left leg forward. Keep your eyes focused ahead while pushing the shoulders down. Return to Step 1 and repeat the exercise in the other direction.

BENEFITS

Spinning in circles is a technique used by warriors to throw their opponents off balance. It increases physical mobility and mental agility. It also unlocks potential vital energy, or *prana,* and focuses the mind to see one spot in each direction without becoming dizzy. The movement should be fluid and continue in one direction before repeating on the other side. The position of the arms can be difficult for some people. Start with the prayer position when both hands are together and place them at the breastbone instead.

Physical
• Increases strength
• Improves energy levels
• Tones arms and legs

Mental
• Promotes positive thinking
• Focuses the mind

Health
• Boosts immune system
• Releases fatigue

Ayurvedic
• Excellent for *Vata* and *Pitta* types

Pranayama

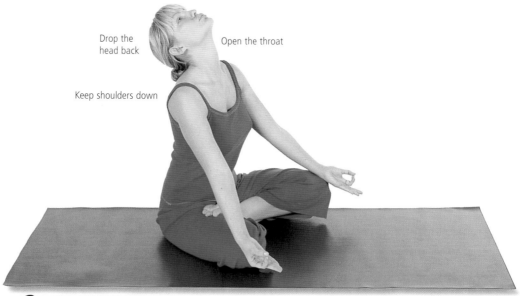

Elbows straight

Straight spine

Thumbs and first
fingers form circles

Tailbone touching the floor

1 Sit up tall in a cross-legged, half lotus, or full lotus position. It is important
that your tailbone touches the floor. Open the palms so they face upward
and hold the thumbs and first fingers together. Keep the remaining fingers
together and rest the back of the hands on the knees. Drop the head
slightly forward and gaze at the fingertips. Inhale deeply through the nose,
and slowly drop the head all the way back.

Drop the
head back

Open the throat

Keep shoulders down

2 Open the mouth to exhale, and make a swooshing sound as you exhale
the breath.

BENEFITS

Pranayama, or the yoga technique of breath control, has many benefits. On the purely physical level, deep breathing increases the oxygen to the system, which then purifies the blood. The cells are replenished and rejuvenated. It also helps balance the left and right hemispheres of the brain, which sends a steady flow of energy through the nervous system. On the mental level, the steady flow of *prana* calms and soothes the brain. When the mind is calm, worries can dissolve and solutions can be found.

Physical
• Increases energy flow
• Improves posture

Mental
• Calms and soothes the brain
• Increases clarity of thought
• Improves concentration

Health
• Purifies blood supply
• Increases lung capacity
• Rejuvenates cells
• Replenishes vital organs
• Promotes a calm and relaxed disposition
• Balances masculine and feminine energies to achieve balance and harmony

Ayurvedic
• Excellent for all *doshas*

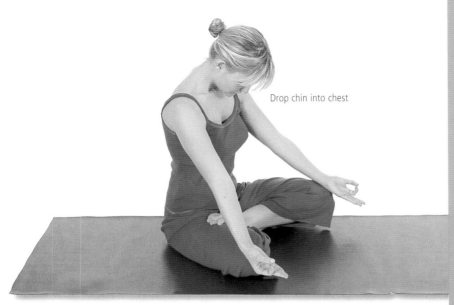

Drop chin into chest

3 Continue to exhale until you drop your chin into the chest.

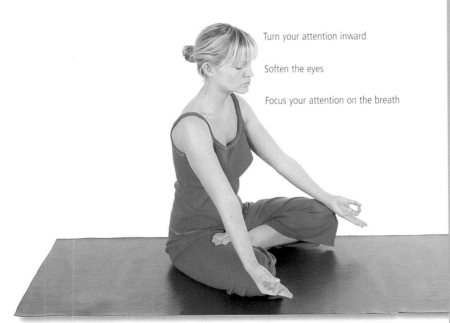

Turn your attention inward

Soften the eyes

Focus your attention on the breath

4 Return to a perfect posture and continue to inhale and exhale through the nose for 10 counts. Keep the breath deep and even. Repeat 5 times.

PRANAYAMA

183

Candle gazing

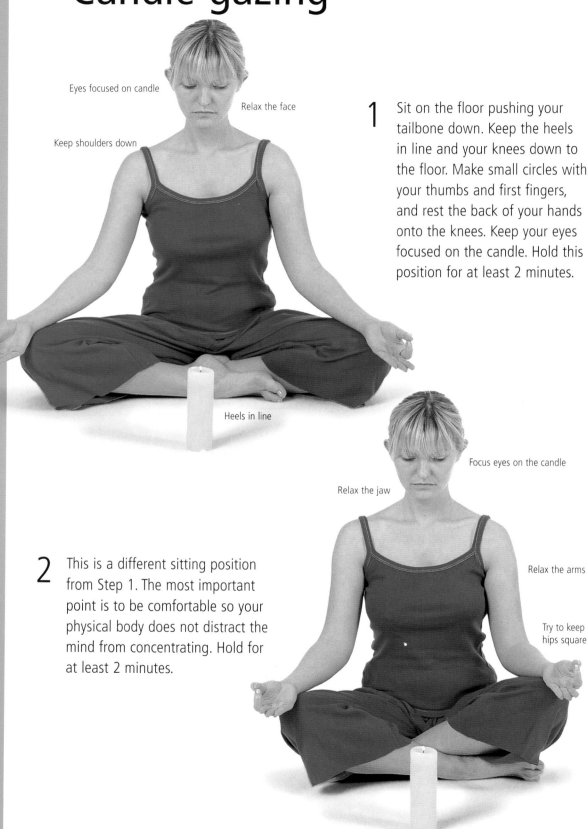

Eyes focused on candle

Relax the face

Keep shoulders down

Heels in line

1 Sit on the floor pushing your tailbone down. Keep the heels in line and your knees down to the floor. Make small circles with your thumbs and first fingers, and rest the back of your hands onto the knees. Keep your eyes focused on the candle. Hold this position for at least 2 minutes.

Focus eyes on the candle

Relax the jaw

Relax the arms

Try to keep hips square

2 This is a different sitting position from Step 1. The most important point is to be comfortable so your physical body does not distract the mind from concentrating. Hold for at least 2 minutes.

BENEFITS

Candle gazing is a technique that trains the mind to concentrate. When you gaze continuously at any object for a few seconds and close your eyes, the image remains briefly. If you gaze steadily at the candle and flame, when you close your eyes, you will see the flame for a moment. Candle gazing trains the mind to retain the light image and keep it there. This symbolizes the white light that is the soul. After continued practice, you will be able to hold the light in your inner vision. With more experience, you will see the light without using a candle. This will help you open the third eye—the inner vision that restores your mind, body, and spiritual self to harmony and balance.

Physical
- Promotes a glowing complexion
- Promotes sparkling eyes

Mental
- Promotes mental calm
- Promotes inner calm
- Promotes positive thinking
- Increases clarity of thought

Health
- Calms nervous system
- Destresses the mind
- Restores harmony and balance
- Cures insomnia
- Cures anxiety
- Unblocks energy centers, preventing disease
- Boosts mental and physical health

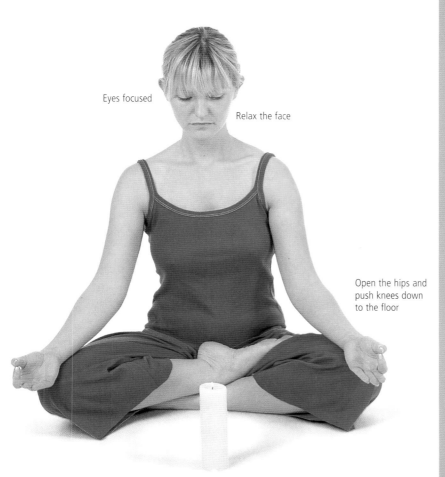

Eyes focused

Relax the face

Open the hips and push knees down to the floor

3 This is the half lotus pose that forces your tailbone to touch the floor while keeping the spine erect. When the spine is totally erect, as in this pose, the energy between the *chakras,* or energy centers are free to travel up through the spine to release any blockages. Hold for at least 2 minutes and build up mental stamina to hold as long as you can.

Visualization

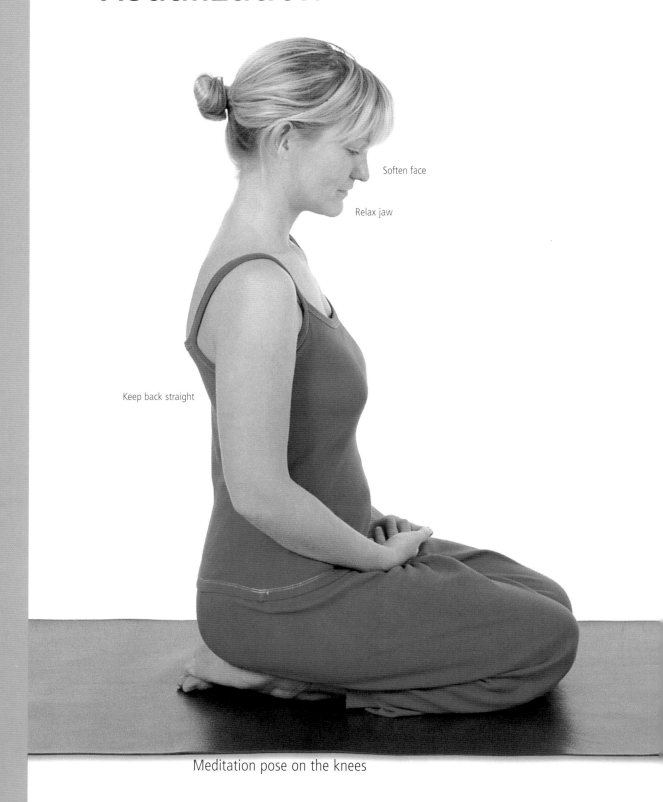

Soften face

Relax jaw

Keep back straight

Meditation pose on the knees

BENEFITS

Visualization helps you to connect to the cosmic force that is the purpose of life. Meditation brings the source of knowledge and wisdom. When you master it, you will find peace, happiness, and serenity. Imagine the energy from the base *chakra*. Feel it move up through the spine up to the crown *chakra* at the top of the head to join with the cosmic energy. It is then that the principles of life become clear and the mind, body, and spiritual Selves are unified.

For another visualization, lie on your back with your knees up, feet flat on the floor, arms at your sides with palms down and eyes open.

To relax after visualization or to help deep sleep, adopt the final pose of Deep relaxation (see page 159), but with your hands, palms together, under your cheek.

Physical
• Promotes radiance and inner beauty

Mental
• Enhances solitude and wisdom
• Promotes inner joy, peace, and harmony
• Increases mental balance

Health
• Reduces stress on all levels
• Enahnces ability for self-healing
• Combats mental illness
• Cures insomnia

Ayurvedic
• The art of visualization is important for all *doshas*

Index

A

abdomen 90
  back twist 106–7
  deep lunge balance 123
  Jet 74–5
  leg kicks 179
  leg lift 60–3
  Locust 94–5
  modified Bow 102–3
  sitting balance 64–7
  spinal twist 151
  standing Bow 136–7
  stomach stretches 90–1
  Warrior 56–7
  Wheel 138–9
  yoga menu 11
accidents, passive yoga 17
aging 97
  face and throat 82
  loss of flexibility 41
  Panchakarma 125
  Rabbit 143
  and weight gain 15, 117
AIDS 15, 19
alcohol 25
anabolism 18
ankles, yoga menu 13
arms
  back bend 58–9
  breathing with arms 98–9
  Circles 180–1
  Dog 144–5
  Letter T 72–3
  one-arm balance 68–71
  push-ups 86–7
  rejuvenation 154–5
  Triangle 52–3
  upper arm flabbiness 86
  Wheel 138–9
  yoga menu 9
arthritis 17, 59, 97
asanas 17, 24
asthma 17
Ayurveda 18–23, 97, 125

B

back
  back bend 58–9
  back twist 106–7
  breathe and relax 78–81
  Camel 88–9
  Cat 104–5
  Cobra 112–13
  Fish 82–3
  flexibility 14
  head rolls 110–11
  Kundalini 17
  leg lift 60–3
  lying flat twist 140–1
  Plough 117
  Rabbit 143
  rejuvenation 155
  side stretch 92–3, 120–1
  sitting balance 64–7
  spinal twist 76–7, 146–51
  standing Bow 136–7
  stiffness 41
  tension in 108
  Triangle 52–3
  Warrior 56–7
  Wheel 138–9
  yoga menu 10
back pain 17, 90, 104
  back bend 59
  back twist 107
  lying flat twist 141
  sitting balance 65
  spinal twist 77, 147
  Triangle 53
  yoga menu 10
balance
  balancing workout 126–33
  deep lunge balance 122–3
  inner balance 14, 124
  loss of 41
  one-arm balance 68–71
  sitting balance 64–7
  Tree 134–5
Bhakti Yoga 16
blood circulation see circulation
body composition 41
Bow
  modified Bow 102–3
  standing Bow 136–7
brain 17
  Pranayama 183
  Rabbit 143
breathing 28–9
  breathe and relax 78–81, 152–3
  breathing with arms 98–9
  deep-breathing exercises 14
  energy booster 100–1
  Kalaripayatt 160
  nerve soother 156–7
  oxygen levels 97, 98, 101
  Pranayama 28, 160, 161, 182–3
  rejuvenation 154
Buddhism 16
buttocks
  balancing workout 127
  Cobra 112–13
  deep lunge balance 123
  Jet 74–5
  Letter T 72–3
  Locust 94–5
  modified Bow 102–3
  rejuvenation 155
  Wheel 138–9
  yoga menu 12

C

Camel 88–9
cancer 15, 19, 41, 96
candle gazing 184–5
cardiorespiratory fitness 41
Cat 104–5
catabolism 18
cellulite 15
chakras 88, 125, 155, 185, 187
chanting 16
chest
  Camel 88–9
  opening 88
  yoga menu 10
Circles 180–1
circulation
  balancing workout 127
  breathe and relax 153
  cardiorespiratory fitness 41
  deep lunge balance 123
  Jet 75
  Letter T 73
  rejuvenation 155
  shoulder stand 114–15
  side stretch 120–1
  Triangle 53
  shoulder stand 114–15
  warm-up 42–51
  yoga menu 10

clothing 24
Cobra 112–13
colon, Warrior 57
concentration
    candle gazing 185
    yoga menu 8
constipation
    sitting balance 65
    Triangle 53
contraindications 25
coordination, loss of 41
Cosmic Universe 16, 161
cramps, menstrual
    Plough 117
    yoga menu 12
cravings 112, 161

D
dancer's pose 137
deep lunge balance 122–3
deep relaxation 158–9
degenerative diseases 97
depression 19, 115, 120
diabetes 41, 96
diaphragm, breathing from 157
digestive system 102
    disorders 97
    sitting balance 65
    spinal twist 77
    Triangle 53
    yoga menu 11
disabled people, passive yoga 17
diseases see illness
dizziness 25
doctors
    Ayurvedic medicine 19
    passive yoga 17
Dog 144–5
doshas, Ayurveda 18–23, 97, 125
drugs 25

E
elbow joint problems 41
    yoga menu 9
elderly people, passive yoga 17
Elephant 174–5
endocrine glands
    balancing workout 127
    see also hormones
endurance 41
energy
    energy booster 100–1
    energy levels 14, 41

Hatha Yoga 16
    prana 28, 125, 153, 159
environment, practising yoga 24
exercise, yoga for 40–95
    back bend 58–9
    breathe and relax 78–81
    Camel 88–9
    Fish 82–3
    Jet 74–5
    leg lift 60–3
    Letter T 72–3
    Locust 94–5
    one-arm balance 68–71
    push-ups 86–7
    shoulder release 84–5
    side stretch 92–3
    sitting balance 64–7
    spinal twist 76–7
    stomach stretches 90–1
    Triangle 52–3
    warm-up 42–51
    Warrior 54–7

F
face
    aging 82
    modified Bow 103
    nerve soother 157
    yoga menu 8
faeces 125
fat
    body composition 41
    cellulite 15
fatigue 120
feet 24
    yoga menu 13
feminine energies 16, 24
fertility problems 112
Fish 82–3
fitness 41
flexibility 41
four paths 16
free radicals 125

G
genetics, illness and 96
God 17
Gyana Yoga 16
gynaecological problems, yoga
    menu 12

H
half lotus pose 185

hamstrings, leg lift 60–3
Hatha Yoga 16, 17
head
    head rolls 110–11
    yoga menu 8
headaches
    Cat 105
    spinal twist 77, 147
    yoga menu 8
health, yoga for 96–123
    back twist 106–7
    breathing with arms 98–9
    Cat 104–5
    Cobra 112–13
    deep lunge balance 122–3
    energy booster 100–1
    head rolls 110–11
    modified Bow 103
    Plough 116–17
    shoulder shrugs 108–9
    shoulder stand 114–15
    side stretch 120–1
heart
    cardiorespiratory fitness 41
    chakra 88
    deep lunge balance 123
    heart disease 15, 19, 41, 96
    Letter T 73
    Rabbit 143
    side stretch 120–1
    Wheel 138–9
    yoga menu 10
Hinduism 16, 17
hips
    back bend 58–9
    breathe and relax 78–81
    rejuvenation 155
    sitting balance 64–7
    spinal twist 76–7, 147
hormones
    balancing workout 127
    benefits of yoga 15
    Plough 117
    shoulder stand 115
    women's problems 112
    yoga menu 8, 11
Horse 172–3
hypertension 157

I
illness 15, 17, 96
    Ayurvedic medicine 19, 125
    cardiorespiratory fitness 41

immune system 15, 97, 125
  Dog 145
  one-arm balance 69
inner balance 14, 124
insomnia, yoga menu 8
intestines, spinal twist 151
inverted postures
  Plough 116–19
  shoulder stand 114–15

J
Jet 74–5
joints
  flexibility 125
  stiffness 41

K
Kalaripayatt 160, 175
Kapha, Ayurveda 18, 19, 23, 125
Karma Yoga 16
kicks, leg 178–9
kidneys 102
  spinal twist 77, 147, 151
  Warrior 57
kneeling posture 27
knees
  stiffness 41
  yoga menu 13
Kundalini Yoga 17

L
legs
  Circles 180–1
  Cobra 112–13
  deep lunge balance 123
  Dog 144–5
  Jet 74–5
  leg kicks 178–9
  leg lift 60–3
  Locust 94–5
  rejuvenation 155
  sitting balance 64–7
  standing Bow 136–7
  Tree 134–5
  Triangle 52–3
  Warrior 54–7
  Wheel 138–9
  yoga menu 13
Letter T 72–3
lifestyle changes 25
Lion 176–7
liver 102
  spinal twist 151

  Warrior 57
Locust 94–5
lotus pose 185
lumbago 90, 104, 107, 141
lungs
  breathe and relax 153
  breathing 28
  breathing with arms 98–9
  Camel 89
  cardiorespiratory fitness 41
  Fish 83
  Letter T 73
lying flat twist 140–1
lymph system
  balancing workout 127
  breathe and relax 153

M
mantras 16
martial arts 160
masculine energies 16, 24
master hormone, yoga menu 8
mats 24
medicines 25
meditation 15, 161
  meditation in motion 162–71
  visualization 186–7
menstrual cramps
  Plough 117
  yoga menu 12
menstrual cycle 115
mental yoga 16
menus 8–13
metabolism 112, 153
  aging 15
  Ayurveda 18
  Plough 116–19
middle-age spread 15, 117
migraine 17
  yoga menu 8
mind and spirit, yoga for 15,
    160–87
  calming the mind 98, 101, 153,
    157, 161
  candle gazing 184–5
  Circles 180–1
  Elephant 174–5
  Horse 172–3
  leg kicks 178–9
  Lion 176–7
  meditation 161
  meditation in motion 162–71
  Pranayama 182–3

  visualization 186–7
  modified Bow 102–3
mood swings 112, 115
Mountain 26
muscles
  fitness 41
  warm-up 42–51
  yoga menu 9

N
nausea 25
neck
  Cobra 112–13
  energy booster 101
  Fish 82–3
  head rolls 110–11
  Jet 74–5
  modified Bow 103
  nerve soother 157
  spinal twist 147
  tension in 84, 108–9
  Wheel 139
  yoga menu 9
nervous system 17, 97
  balancing workout 127
  breathe and relax 153
  Dog 145
  nerve injuries 17
  nerve soother 156–7
  Pranayama 161, 183
  Rabbit 143
  sitting balance 65
Nirvana 16
nostrils, breathing 28–9

O
one-arm balance 68–71
osteoporosis 97
ovaries 112
oxygen
  rejuvenation 154
  shoulder stand 114–15
  see also breathing

P
pain
  loss of flexibility 41
  neck and shoulder 108
  see also back pain
Panchakarma 125
pancreas 65
panic attacks 17, 157
parathyroid glands 83

passive yoga 17
pectoral muscles, yoga menu 10
pelvic region, yoga menu 12
peptic ulcers 96
physical yoga 16–17
pineal gland 83
Pitta, Ayurveda 18, 19, 21, 125
pituitary gland 83
Plough 116–19
pollution 25
posture 26–7
practising yoga 24–5
Prakruti 18
prana 28, 98, 125, 153, 159
Pranayama 28–9, 98, 154, 160, 161, 182–3
prayer 16
pregnancy
    contraindications for yoga 25
    fertility problems 112
    yoga menu 12
purification 125
push-ups 86–7

Q
Queen's pose 115

R
Rabbit 142–3
Raj Yoga 16, 17
rejuvenation 125, 154–5
relaxation 15, 17
    breathe and relax 78–81, 152–3
    deep relaxation 158–9
relevance of yoga 17
respiration *see* breathing

S
salute to the sun 30–9
sciatica 90, 104
    back twist 107
    lying flat twist 141
    sitting balance 65
    Triangle 53
Self, purpose of yoga 14, 16
self-esteem 120
senility 143
shoulders
    back bend 58–9
    energy booster 101
    Fish 82–3

head rolls 110–11
nerve soother 157
shoulder release 84–5
shoulder shrugs 108–9
shoulder stand 114–15
spinal twist 147
stiffness 41
tension in 108–9
yoga menu 9
side stretch 92–3, 120–1
sitting balance 64–7
sitting posture 27
    candle gazing 184–5
skin disorders 19
sleep problems, yoga menu 8
smoking 25
Soul 15
spine *see* back
spinning in circles 180–1
spirit *see* mind and spirit
spleen 102
    spinal twist 77
    Warrior 57
stamina 14
    cardiorespiratory fitness 41
standing Bow 136–7
standing posture 26
static poses, Warrior 54–7
stiff neck, yoga menu 9
stomach *see* abdomen
strength 14, 41
stress-relief, yoga for 124–59
    balancing workout 126–33
    benefits of 15, 17, 41
    breathe and relax 152–3
    deep relaxation 158–9
    Dog 144–5
    lying flat twist 140–1
    nerve soother 156–7
    Rabbit 143
    rejuvenation 154–5
    standing Bow 136–7
    Tree 134–5
    Wheel 138–9
    yoga menu 8
stretching, benefits of 14, 41
sweat 125

T
Tadasana 26
tendons, stiffness 41
tension, in neck and shoulders 84, 108–9

thighs
    yoga menu 13
    see also legs
third eye 185
throat, aging 82
thyroid gland 112, 115
toxins 25, 28, 97, 102, 125, 147
Tree 134–5
Triangle 52–3
twists
    back twist 106–7
    lying flat twist 140–1
    spinal twist 76–7, 146–51
    Warrior 56–7

U
Universal Cosmos 16
urinary disorders 97
urine 125
uterus 112

V
Vata, Ayurveda 18, 20, 125
Vedanta 16
Vedas 14, 18
Vikrruti 18
visualization 15, 17, 186–7

W
waist
    balancing workout 127
    side stretch 92–3
    yoga menu 10
warm-up 42–51
Warrior 54–7
waste products 125
weight control 15, 41, 112, 115, 117
Wheel 138–9
whiplash injury, yoga menu 9
women's problems 112
wrists
    back bend 58–9
    yoga menu 9

Y
yogis 161

Acknowledgments

Executive Editor: Jane McIntosh
Editorial Director: Jane Birch
Editor: Cathy Lowne
Executive Art Editor: Rozelle Bentheim
Design: Maggie Town and Beverly Price
Picture Research: Jennifer Veall
Senior Production Controller: Jo Sim
Photography: Peter Pugh-Cook

Vimla Lalvani studied dance under the great masters Martha Graham and Merce Cunningham and went on to become the personal student of one of the most influential figures in yoga today, B.K.S. Iyengar. An acknowledged authority and acclaimed yoga teacher, Vimla has made many television appearances and has produced a number of best-selling videos and successful books.